MW01678885

Toxic Food Syndrome

95 out of 100 people are poisoning themselves and don't even know it!

Are you one of them?

This is a body of work representing 27 years of activity and service. Names and places of patients have been changed by the author to protect and respect their privacy. All stories are true, based upon letters, audio or video recordings received from the people themselves, their healthcare professionals or from televised shows.

Cover design by Ann Schneider

First printing February 2002
Second printing September 2002
Third printing May 2003
Fourth printing January 2004
Fifth printing June 2004
Sixth printing January 2005
Seventh printing September 2005

"115,000 copies now in print"

For information, address: Fun Publishing
6801 Powerline Road, Fort Lauderdale, FL 33309

ISBN 0-9718802-6-3

To Cher, Chele and David—
my inspiring family. Thank you for your
support as I continue to dedicate so much of
my time to this work. I'm deeply grateful for
your helping me prove within our own lives—
beyond any doubt—that the right food is truly
your first and best medicine.

Acknowledgments

I would like to thank the thousands of physicians worldwide who have entrusted Immuno Laboratories to provide consistently reliable, clinically useful testing. We never take your trust or loyalty for granted.

I would also like to thank a wide spectrum of our physicians' patients ages 2-82. Your precious, miracle-like stories of better health and healing have been documented in letter, email, fax, audio and video mediums. Your results fuel our desire to spread the word on this exciting way to help others.

My deepest gratitude goes to my parents. You have always supported my quest for insights into health optimization and you have dedicated and sacrificed your time to help me create this service.

I wish to thank the entire staff of Immuno Laboratories for making it possible to share this amazing 27-year story. Working as a team, you have the proud legacy of helping tens of thousands of people who now live healthier and happier lives.

I want to acknowledge my mentors who, at one point or another in my life, were powerful positive influences on my personal growth and development: Martin Stern,

Ivan Popov, M.D., Elliot Goldwag, Ph.D., Doug Kaufmann, David Wallack, and Sydney Klein—thank you!

Contents

Introduction

If you are like 95 percent of the population, you are poisoning yourself every day.

There is an old saying that some people live to eat, while others eat to live. But the tragic fact is most people are actually eating to die—or at least exist in a sort of living death.

Stop right now and think about it. When was the last time you made an excuse for something in your body that hurt, or when you simply lacked the energy to get up and go. Does the phrase, "I must be getting older," sound all-too familiar? Or how about, "After 40, it's all downhill from there." What health problems have you simply learned to live with, while telling yourself, your family and others you are getting old?

Well, I have news for you about this old age stuff. In 1999, Franklin Mason of Mullins, S.C., ran the Grandfather Mountain Marathon not far from where I was living and writing this book. He covered the 26.2 miles, all up and down some of the steepest parts of the Appalachians, in 4 hours, 57 minutes and 31 seconds. What makes that amazing is he was 74 years old, and running a mile every 11.3 minutes! But wait—there is more to the story. Mr.

Mason was back in 2000, but didn't finish quite as fast: it took him 5 hours, 1 minute and 6 seconds (at age 75) to cover one of the toughest courses anywhere. There's more: he came back in 2001 and beat his record for the past two years, finishing in just 4:53:06—at age 76.

Or consider Edith Autorino, who in 2000 completed the Ironman Triathlon in Hawaii. She swam 2.4 miles, bicycled 112 miles and ran 26.2 miles—and did it all in a record (for her age group) of 15 hours, 19 minutes and 20 seconds. Not bad for someone 70 years old.

So what gives? Here you are, nursing aches and pains and minor ailments all the time, and these folks are out running marathons when they are your age, or 10, 20, 30, 40 or even 50 years older. The answer is a secret I learned the hard way, but I want you to learn the easy way: many of the chronic conditions that are limiting you and taking the enjoyment out of your life are the direct result of what you eat. I'm not talking about food that is not nutritious; I'm talking about everyday foods, which are toxic to your particular system. **Each of us is an individual, with particular nutritional needs, and we're unknowingly eating foods that are toxic to us.**

I'm not talking about food that is not nutritious; I'm talking about everyday foods, which are toxic to your particular system.

Anyone who has enjoyed the movie "Mrs. Doubtfire" will remember the scene where Robin Williams slips Pierce Brosnan some pepper, knowing he'd have a toxic reaction to it. In a few seconds, Brosnan's character is gasping for breath. That sort of food toxicity is obvious and dramatic. But most toxic reactions to foods are subtle and show up in ways that the victims—including you—overlook or excuse.

Put another way: Brosnan's reaction to that pepper was acute—violent, sudden and life-threatening. But as you will learn in this book, most toxic reactions to food are subtle, long-lasting and life-damaging.

Take the case of Sydney Mackey. She suffered from food toxicities and asthma practically from birth. At age 3, her family moved to Arizona in a desperate effort to improve her health. Even so, she was hospitalized at least once a year for the next five years. Sydney was constantly sick and took lots and lots of antibiotics. If she stopped taking them, she immediately developed colds, which then turned into bronchitis and sinus infections. As an adult, after having a food toxicity test, she redesigned her diet with the help of her doctor. "Within two weeks I felt so much better it was hard to believe," she said. "Symptoms disappeared that I hadn't even been aware of: various aches and pains I considered normal." When her kids brought home colds, she was able to fight them off for the first time in her life.

What did that test show? Sydney's system showed quite a few toxic food reactions to over 100 foods for which she was tested.

Food toxicities lie behind many chronic conditions. And here's some more news: chronic conditions are the biggest challenge people and the medical profession face.

Medical spending in the United States now exceeds $1.2 trillion annually. Of that, 75 percent is spent on chronic conditions, those ailments—the migraine headaches, arthritis, hyperactivity, ear infections, excess weight, irritable bowel, psoriasis and other symptoms—you wish would just go away. An overwhelming majority of the 2.9 billion prescriptions physicians write each year are to help people deal with chronic problems.

An overwhelming majority of the 2.9 billion prescriptions physicians write each year are to help people deal with chronic problems.

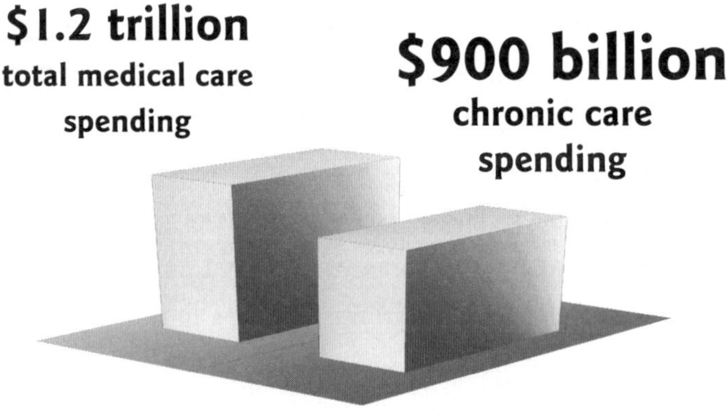

Many treatments of chronic conditions only treat the symptoms and suppress them. That's what happened to Sydney Mackey: her doctors tried to control her symptoms, but never found the underlying source of her problem.

Now imagine if you had a car, and the engine missed all the time. You went to a mechanic, and he couldn't find the problem. Then to another mechanic, and she couldn't find the problem. Then, you discovered your fuel was contaminated with water—regular, plain old water. Add a little to the highest-octane fuel and the newest, most powerful engine will knock, stall and maybe quit running entirely. That is because internal combustion engines burn only a certain type of fuel, and you might say they are toxically reactive to any other kind. **Think about that**—water is essential to our lives and toxic to your automobile engine!

Your body is something like that engine. It takes fuel—food and water—and runs on it. And, just like that engine, you put things in your body it cannot tolerate, it will begin to "knock" and "stall." Your body's "mechanics" (one or more medical doctors) may not recognize the source of your problems. After a while, many people who suffer from chronic conditions look for help beyond conventional medicine. Some physicians even recommend certain of these treatments. Statistics show that 60 percent of patients are now taking alternatives and most never tell their doctors. That is potentially dangerous, because the medical doctor may prescribe medicines that could have interactions with these alternative treatments.

Statistics show that 60 percent of patients are now taking alternatives and most never tell their doctors.

The ultimate alternative, I've found, is not in a medicine bottle. The ultimate alternative is the food you eat! The truth is eating the wrong food can be devastating; eating the right food is truly your first and best medicine.

I call what happens to people—including me—when they eat the wrong foods Toxic Food Syndrome, TFS for short. TFS can ruin a person's life.

Take the case of the Winston family. When their daughter Jane was three, she started having constant stomach aches and fevers. When she turned four, the pain became so bad Jane would scream and cry in pain. The best diagnosis a medical doctor could suggest was the little girl chewed too much gum.

By the time she was five, Jane was constantly agitated and frustrated—and still in pain. As young as she was, Jane was depressed, and even talked of killing herself and her family. She said she heard voices in her head. In fits of rage, she would destroy her room and punch holes in walls.

"All the doctors we had gone to told us it was all in her mind," recalls her mother, Mary Winston. "We were so frustrated we almost decided to put her in a foster home; our lives were a mess. We couldn't handle her fits three and four times a day."

Then, finally, the Wintons took Jane to a physician who recommended she have a food toxicity test. The little girl showed toxic reactions to 25 foods. In just one month, all the pain, rage and seeming mental illness was gone. "If it wasn't for this great test my daughter would be in foster care or a mental home for the rest of her life," Mrs. Winston said. A life could have been wasted—because of TFS!

"If it wasn't for this great test my daughter would be in foster care or a mental home for the rest of her life."

After hearing these stories, you will want to start eating right. The problem is: what's right for you? One expert will recommend high protein, low carbohydrate; another expert literally recommends the exact opposite, low protein, high complex carbohydrate; and yet another expert recommends vegetarian or macrobiotic food plans. What's right for you? That is where toxic food testing comes in. One simple blood test will reveal the foods that are virtual poison to your particular system and other foods that will more readily be digested, assimilated and used by your body to produce more energy and well being, helping you chart the path to improved health.

Obesity is a global disease—it's virtually an epidemic. Fad diets, diet drinks, appetite suppressors, fat blockers, surgical procedures and other products make the weight control industry a multi-billion dollar enterprise with everyone's failed attempts to lose pounds and maintain their desired weight. Ever wonder why diets don't work? You're about to learn the secret to successful dieting. As you read through this book, you will discover how toxic food testing makes every diet work better, simply by showing you which foods in your chosen diet are the right ones for you and, most importantly, which foods in your diet are virtual poison.

Just one more important fact before we take an in-depth look at how conquering Toxic Food Syndrome can change your life: Today, medical doctors and other healthcare providers all over the world have become qualified providers of the Immuno 1 Bloodprint™, a food toxicity test. Each one can tell remarkable stories of patients whose lives were turned around when they found out the food they were eating was ruining their lives—often times just a few everyday foods.

You're probably spending thousands of dollars on foods each year that are unknowingly virtual poison to your system. This book will show you how to save money by making the right food your first and best medicine. As you continue to read this book, you are going on an exciting adventure of discovery. In these pages, you will learn about what is really happening inside you—how the food you are eating may well be at the root of your health problems—and how you can change your life completely, just by understanding what Toxic Food Syndrome can do, and is doing to you. Armed with this knowledge, you can win your battle for better health and save tons of money not having to replenish your supply of over the counter remedies, reduce doctor visits, expensive prescription medicines and choose delicious foods that your particular system will properly digest and assimilate.

<u>A modest example:</u>

Medication	$600/year
Lost work days	$300/year
Grocery dollars spent on foods causing toxic reactions	20% of $6000 or $1200
Yearly losses	$2100/year
Lifetime losses	$63,000 or more!

<u>Now it's your turn to fill in the blanks:</u>

Your medication costs	?
Your lost workday costs	?
Your grocery dollars spent on foods causing toxic reactions	?
Your total cash losses over a lifetime of your disease	?

How much is your disease costing you?

Chapter 1

An estimated 95 percent of the population suffers from Toxic Food Syndrome.

If you are suffering from Toxic Food Syndrome, believe me, you are not alone.

An estimated 95 percent of the population suffers from Toxic Food Syndrome. The symptoms vary from individual to individual, but all have one thing in common: when a person stops eating the foods that are causing toxic reactions in their particular system, their symptoms disappear. These symptoms range from indigestion to earaches to stomach aches to joint pain, to extremes of what might be considered mental illness.

For most people, however, TFS means a range of annoying but not life-threatening symptoms to which they have adapted their lives. That's right: they have made a peace of sorts with Toxic Food Syndrome, accepting aches, pains, discomfort, lack of energy and more as a way of life. Be honest: haven't you done the same thing?

That backache that makes you not want to get out of bed in the morning could well be the result of the lunch you ate the day before. Your indigestion you call having a "sensitive stomach" may be sensitive—but only to certain foods that are toxic to your system.

Wouldn't you rather feel great every morning? Wouldn't you like to enjoy life to its fullest? If you could, would you trim 20 years off your age? I bet you would—and now you can, by eliminating all those "age-related" problems that really stem from one source: Toxic Food Syndrome.

Let me stress something, however: Toxic Food Syndrome is not a disease that only affects adults. There are millions of children, and yours may be among them, for whom life is a living hell because of toxic food. Jan Kohl's 21-month-old daughter was diagnosed with a reflux disorder that threatened kidney and other damage. She was put on antibiotics, and life became a succession of yeast and bladder infections. Her behavior became worse and worse. Jan recalls, "a relative even asked us if she'd been diagnosed with ADHD and how early could they put kids on Ritalin! She never stopped moving, she had no attention span, she was moody, she was clumsy, she made us despair of our abilities as parents." That's some life for a toddler, isn't it?

Fortunately, her parents weren't willing to accept that kind of life for their daughter. They took her to doctors, they researched on the Internet and then they took her to a physician who had the child take the Immuno 1 Bloodprint™. When the test results came back, the family learned their little daughter was suffering from eating 18 foods causing toxic reactions to her particular system. She stopped eating those foods, and what happened was nothing short of a miracle.

"Within two weeks we noticed a dramatic difference," Jan's mom told us in a letter. "Her bladder problems and yeast infections were gone." She was sleeping through the night for the first time, and, as an unexpected bonus her personality changed completely. Don't misunderstand, we loved our daughter, but it was a blessing to see to her go from church nursery terror to a sweet, gentle happy little girl ... almost overnight she was calm, sweet, affectionate and responded to discipline for the first time. What started as a search for help with her reflux disorder became the start of a whole new life for her family. None of us realized how much stress her problems were causing us all."

She added one more thought: "I shudder to think how many children her age are drugged to solve a problem that could be as simple as changing their diet." I shudder at that thought, too. What was this little girl's future if her parents hadn't discovered toxic food reactions were at the root of her problems? A lifetime of unnecessary medication, "special" classes in school, constant discipline problems, and years spent in physical misery. Trust me, she is not alone. Maybe when you read Jan's story, you recognize your own family and children.

"I shudder to think how many children her age are drugged to solve a problem that could be as simple as changing their diet."

One point she made is how much her daughter's problems impacted the whole family. Think how your "little" health problems are affecting your family. Dad doesn't have much energy after supper, so there is no one to play ball with the kids. A camping or hiking adventure would have been great—10 years ago. Mom's "bad stomach" makes it hard to want to do much of anything. **There is enough pressure on families today from many sources without having to deal with chronic pain and fatigue.**

TFS – My Own Story

How do I know so much about Toxic Food Syndrome? Because I am among the 95 percent of the population that suffers from TFS. If you are suffering from TFS, I can feel for you because I have been there. Let me tell you my story.

This book was actually started *before* I was born. My mother was sick to her stomach every night of her pregnancy with me. As I think back, her sickness probably programmed me to have sensitive digestion before I even left her womb. I have struggled with toxic food reactions all my life. Of course, no physician ever interpreted it that way. My otitis media (inner ear infections), periodic episodes of diarrhea and constipation, and endless stomachaches were treated as individual symptoms—never seen as some sort of pattern or syndrome. And, of course, many of my symptoms were treated with repeated courses of antibiotics.

From the time I could ride a bicycle until my high school years, my breakfasts consisted of riding to the nearby bakery and picking up fresh jellyrolls and white breakfast rolls for my brother, parents and I. I'd eat one of each of these rolls and washed it down with hot chocolate. I'm glad I'm still alive and in reasonably good health in spite of such poor dietary habits!

"From the time I could ride a bicycle until my high school years, my breakfasts consisted of riding to the nearby bakery and picking up fresh jellyrolls and white breakfast rolls for my brother, parents and I."

It wasn't until I graduated high school and entered college that I ever learned anything about the link between what I was eating and how I was feeling. Gradually, in Madison, Wisconsin—a campus of 30,000 students at that time—I made new friends who were "health nuts," buying organic food from cooperatives, eating dried seaweed, fasting, cleansing, and even some strict vegetarians. For the first time, I was meeting people who felt deeply about their diets and the impact what they ate had on how they felt.

This triggered my lifelong interest in the power of food. I experimented throughout my college years with just a variety of diets popular at the time: raw foods, lacto-vegetarian, strict vegetarian, and lots of fasting using fresh, raw juices. Each of these experiments proved to have merit, but none of them completely resolved my delicate digestive system. I felt better, but not consistently healthy.

After graduating college, I was soon provided a unique opportunity to manage a very innovative holistic longevity center, Renaissance Revitalization Center in Nassau, Bahamas. I pursued a more balanced Bahamian diet of fish, vegetables and grains. This diet proved to be one of the better diets for me. But, more important, it was here, in the Bahamas that I learned about toxic food testing.

Renaissance was such an innovative facility; it attracted celebrities and other innovative scientists and doctors interested in working with us and always arriving to share their novel insights into health and well-being. One such American scientist introduced me to the notion of toxic food testing. His method, now outdated by newer technology, involved a microscopic observation of your blood cells, which were exposed to food extracts. Toxic food reactions could be observed as the blood cells burst open and were easily observed with the aid of the microscope. I learned this method and returned to the United States to attempt to offer this testing to physicians in my area.

I met with immediate success and found that nearly every person I tested had remarkable results with a wide variety of chronic unresolved symptoms and conditions. Imagine my delight after suffering so many years with what I now know to be toxic reactions to foods and discovering a test that would save one time and suffering by identifying toxic foods.

I launched my laboratory on the kitchen table of my parent's condominium and over time it slowly grew to become a licensed medical laboratory with offices located in Fort Lauderdale, Florida.

"The number of tests should really be millions when you measure the value of the information we provide."

Today, my laboratory enjoys a reputation for being the finest toxic food-testing laboratory in the world. We have performed over 250,000 tests through a network of physicians in more than 24 different countries. The number of tests should really be millions when you measure the value of the information we provide. But, we have continued as an independently owned laboratory using only a small portion of the funds that our testing generates to spread the word.

I do hope that the benefits you receive from your own toxic food test will serve to inspire you to help spread the word about this important test. Please tell your family and friends about the benefits of this testing and help to reduce the number who are suffering needlessly and unknowingly because they simply don't know which foods are the right foods for their particular system.

Most of my adult lifetime has been spent on a single crusade—spreading a simple important message to physicians and the public at large: The right food is your first and best medicine. Now, there's a fast, simple cost effective way to know which food is the right food for you.

The right food is your first and best medicine.

But don't just take my word for it. Immuno Laboratories provided a grant to three medical professionals to conduct a randomized, double blind pilot study of people who reported suffering a variety of symptoms, such as fatigue, hyperactivity, headache, and bowel complaints.

Dr. Sidney MacDonald Baker, M.D., Maureen McDonnell, R.N., and Dr. Carroll V. Truss, Professor Emeritus at the University of Miami, Florida, conducted the study. Their conclusion: eliminating foods our test shows are toxic reduces the symptoms of patients. The study states, "The results of this pilot study support the hypothesis that subjects avoiding IgG reactive (i.e., toxic) foods experience significantly greater symptom relief than subjects avoiding placebo foods." There's more: "The symptoms of subjects responding to dietary manipulation included non-atopic symptoms and, as such, suggest the possibility that symptoms other than those cited in authoritative medical texts may result from food intolerance..."

Immuno Laboratories has spent 27 years improving people's lives. Let's look at some of their stories.

Chapter 2

27 Years, 250,000 Success Stories

Immuno Laboratories has helped people battle Toxic Food Syndrome for 27 years—and there have been a lot of victories along the way.

Each year, many people share their stories with us, writing about the difference conquering Toxic Food Syndrome has made in their lives. I want to share some of the stories with you because I think you will see yourself. Most importantly, you will learn two things: you are not alone in suffering from Toxic Food Syndrome, and there is hope. One day you can be symptom-free, even if you have suffered from TFS for decades.

Children

Let's start with the children.

"Friday, October 17, 1997 was a star spangled day for my ten year old daughter, Mia," wrote Missy Kolson. "She ran off the school bus and announced she had been pain free for the entire day!" Her mother tells what life was like for Mia: "She has been suffering from stomach pain, headaches and swollen joints for, at least, the last two years." Imagine spending two years of your childhood in pain—every day. "We have visited many physicians and have had numerous tests done," Missy wrote. "None had shed any light on her condition. A neighbor who was familiar with your work recommended your laboratory to us. With our pediatrician's assistance, Mia's blood work was sent for testing. Her food sensitivity was a surprise to us all. It is wonderful, as a parent, to finally be able to do something to help alleviate her symptoms. Thanks to the results from your laboratory, we have modified her diet and have seen immediate positive results. We have also witnessed a relapse of swollen knees as soon as she ate something she wasn't supposed to eat."

"Her food sensitivity was a surprise to us all. It is wonderful, as a parent, to finally be able to do something to help alleviate her symptoms."

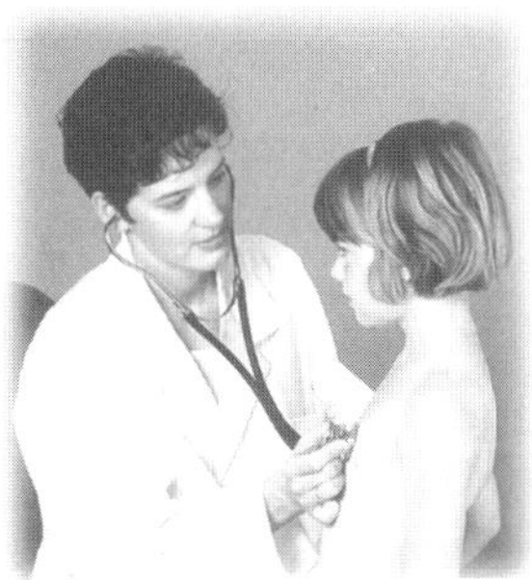

I don't know about you, but thinking about that little girl celebrating her first pain-free day in two years brings tears to my eyes. It's stories like hers that make my lifelong work so special and important to me.

Little David Kaplan (his family calls him "Dak" for short) was a beautiful 10-pound baby when he was born in 1991. He seemed completely healthy until he was eight months old and got a double ear infection. For the next three years, it was one ear infection after another, and one prescription of antibiotics after another. "About 10 days after finishing his prescription we'd be back at the doctor's office again with another ear infection," Dak's mom, Pam, wrote us.

Nothing seemed to stop the ear infections. Dak did not know there was another way of life. "He never complained of symptoms when getting sick," Pam wrote. "He'd be congested for a time, then would cough, spike a fever, get that rheumy look in his eyes and be obviously very ill. It was awful."

When he was five, Dak had an Immuno I Bloodprint™. The results showed these foods caused toxic reactions to him: wheat, dairy, beef, peanuts, crab, lobster, and sesame. "Once he stopped eating the dairy, wheat, etc. his congestion, coughing and other symptoms disappeared!" she wrote. "We just got through the first entire winter of Dak's short little life with no ear infections! What an absolute treat! I go into his room at night and just listen to him breathe—mouth closed, through his nose, no wheezing or coughing—it's heavenly."

We just got through the first entire winter of Dak's short little life with no ear infections! What an absolute treat! I go into his room at night and just listen to him breathe—mouth closed, through his nose, no wheezing or coughing – it's heavenly.

Autism

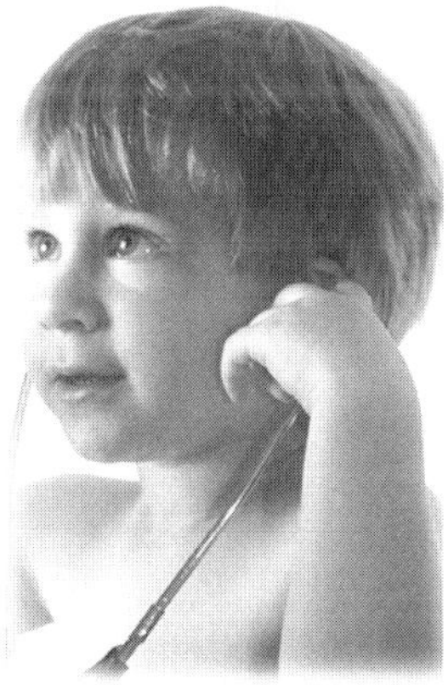

Autism is a devastating condition that affects children. They begin life normally, then gradually withdraw into themselves. In extreme cases, they cannot respond to love and interact better with objects than humans. Tragically, there is no cure. But we hear of cases where autistic children improve when they stop eating toxic foods.

"Last summer, we changed our 4 year old autistic son's diet after testing," wrote Janet L. Presson, R.N. "Within days, Robby became calmer, happier and more focused. He has almost completely stopped spinning and is learning more quickly than ever. As an R.N., I've never seen such profound changes in a child without the use of drugs."

Ramona Delongi wrote, "We are so pleased with the change in our 4 (almost 5) year old son since we found out about his food sensitivities. Having a special needs child we wanted and do want to do all we can. His behavior is more calm and his attention span and eye contact are better. "Mark, our son, is doing quite better in school and (is) beginning to make some sounds. With his autism he is pretty much nonverbal. This is one of the best things we could have done."

"We are so pleased with the change in our 4 (almost 5) year old son since we found out about his food sensitivities. Having a special needs child we wanted and do want to do all we can. His behavior is more calm and his attention span and eye contact are better."

Consider the case of Mickey. He was diagnosed as autistic. He started speaking late, and his speech was limited. He would never look anyone in the eye, which is common in people suffering from autism. When Mickey's mother asked him a question, he would repeat the same question back to her. When he did speak, he always referred to himself in the third person. Here were some more of his traits:

- Mickey would often disappear and worry everyone;
- He would hide in the closet when angry;
- He would often sit alone in the corner of a room;
- He rarely acknowledged or played with his brother;
- He often had fits, at times banging his head against a wall or violently pulling his hair when frustrated;
- He would become so hyperactive that his mother described it as "bouncing off the walls;"
- He often lacked fear in the face of real danger;
- When his mom moved furniture, he felt compelled to move it back to its original place;

- Mickey would frequently spin his whole body around extremely fast, out of control, eventually crashing to the floor;
- He was hypersensitive to sound as if some sounds, such as a lawnmower, were painful to his ears.
- When asked his name or who he was, Mickey never gave his name.

At first, doctors offered no hope. "Don't wait for miracles," one told the family.

What happened next was not a miracle—it was simply that Mickey's family learned the secret that the food you eat is the best medicine possible. In addition to toxic food testing, another type of Bloodprint showed he suffered a systemic yeast infection. A medical doctor prescribed an anti-yeast medication, an anti-yeast diet and had the child avoid all food dyes.

What happened next was not a miracle—it was simply that Mickey's family learned the secret that the food you eat is the best medicine possible.

For the first 10 days, Mickey actually got worse, a result of the destruction of the yeast in his body. But then, two months after eliminating toxic foods from his diet and three months after being treated for a yeast infection, Mickey began to improve in an amazing variety of ways:

- He started concentrating and focusing much better;

- His teachers reported he was consistently doing great;
- Mickey began teasing his parents and brother, something he had never done before;
- He shows signs of having much more fun and acknowledges his brother;
- He rode his bicycle in a parade and won a trophy;
- When asked his name at the parade, the boy responded, "My name is Mickey."

Yes, Mickey is still autistic—but his life has improved dramatically, thanks to this test.

I'm not going to pull any punches when I talk about Attention Deficit Hyperactive Disorder (ADHD) and its milder form, ADD. Hyperactivity is a living hell for those who have it. One 10-year-old boy summed up what it is like to have ADHD when he said, "You wouldn't want to be inside my head. You'd be trampled to death."

Hyperactivity is not a childhood disease that goes away. Children with ADHD grow up to be adults with ADHD. That's a real tragedy, because one study at a federal prison determined that 75 percent of the inmate population had a history of childhood hyperactivity.

"One 10-year-old boy summed up what it is like to have ADHD when he said, "You wouldn't want to be inside my head. You'd be trampled to death."

That doesn't mean your hyperactive child is Public Enemy #1 in the making. What it does mean is that our school system is not set up to deal with kids suffering from ADHD. Simply put, their behaviors—which they cannot help without treatment—irritate other children and drive teachers wild. Hyperactive kids are eight times more likely to drop out than average. A bad school experience can set a child up for a lifetime of failure—or can turn a child into a driven workaholic. The real tragedy is the answer to all this is sitting right in front of the child, on his or her plate.

For many families, the answer has been Ritalin, a powerful drug with many side effects. Frankly, the "cure" can almost be as bad as the disease for the child and their family.

This is not really news. In 1985, the prestigious British medical journal "The Lancet" published a study by Dr. Joseph Egger, head of a pediatric university hospital in Munich, Germany, and another researcher from the Hospital for Sick Children in London. In this study, the two doctors found when they eliminated foods that commonly cause toxic reactions to humans from the diet of hyperactive children, 79 percent of them immediately improved. Subsequent studies have found similar rates of improvement.

The key element missing in this research, however, was determining exactly what foods are toxic to a particular child. That is where the Immuno I Bloodprint™ comes in. By identifying the unique toxic foods for an individual, it paves the way for quick improvements in these cases.

...when they eliminated foods that commonly cause toxic reactions to humans from the diet of hyperactive children, 79 percent of them immediately improved.

Finally, it is hard to put a limit on the kind of problems toxic food reactions can cause in children. "George's skin has cleared up, when before his entire body was red and inflamed with rash—itchy rash," wrote his mom, Cathy. "He is sleeping through most nights and his mommy is too! George's is able to play with his big sister and sometimes even by himself. Before testing, he would sit alone and scratch himself raw if someone wasn't watching him. He is much happier now. It's wonderful to see him walk with a spring in his step while singing to himself." That's what childhood should be like—and can be when you help your child conquer Toxic Food Syndrome.

Headaches

"I immediately stopped eating the food I was reactive to, went on a rotation diet, and have been migraine free for over one and a half years."

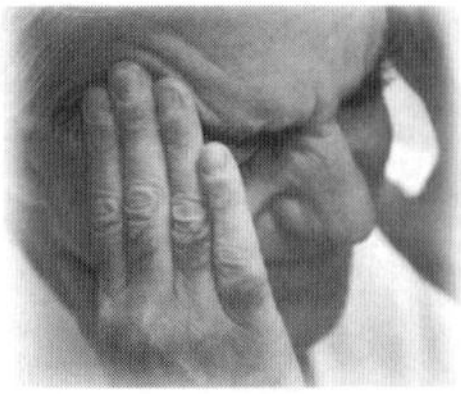

If you have never had a migraine headache, it is hard to explain to you how painful it is. Take a regular headache and multiply the pain many times over. Make it last for days or weeks. That will give you an idea of how painful and crippling migraines can be.

Onami Paj suffered from migraines for 25 years. She wrote she tried, "all sorts of medications to help me get through the day or just to knock me out because the pain was so excruciating. The headaches were sometimes so unbearable that I had to go to the emergency department of my local hospital."

Onami had no relief until she tried an Immuno I Bloodprint™, and learned she was reactive to 21 foods. "I immediately stopped eating the food I was reactive to, went on a rotation diet, and have been migraine free for over one and a half years. I feel reborn and healthy. The quality of my life has changed so drastically that instead of looking forward to two or three painless days a week, I can actually plan on every day being wonderful and pain free."

Does that sound like you? And, like Onami, have you forced yourself to live with migraines or other painful, life-damaging symptoms? Don't assume there is no hope. Consider the case of Urja Isabeli. "Prior to the rotation diet, I've lived with migraine headaches, a stuffy nose, excess mucous, rashes, achy joints, uncontrollable cravings and food binges, colitis, feeling bloated yet constantly hungry, feeling exhausted, depressed and anxious," she wrote us. All this led to a horrible three months of debilitating migraine headaches. Then came the Bloodprint.

Urja learned she had over 20 food toxicities, including some of her favorites, which she ate every day. Soon, she realized they were not "treats" but toxic—at least to her. Fortunately, she took action on this information.

"Once I began the (rotation) diet, I felt relief within three days," Urja wrote. "I was no longer fatigued and anxious I didn't feel bloated or hungry. I haven't had a headache since, I'm no longer stiff on awakening, I've lost 24 pounds, and I'm now living my dream of eating nutritiously and healthy without feeling deprived."

She added something else, "I'm only disappointed that this information isn't more well known and respected by the medical community at large. I could have been saved years of suffering."

Fortunately, it was several years ago when Urja wrote us. Today, medical doctors and other healthcare professionals worldwide are qualified providers of the Immuno I Bloodprint™. Through their highly trained eyes, they can see how the Bloodprint opens the door to a new way of life for their patients.

Like Dorothy Crowch. When she first heard of the Bloodprint, she was 30-something, weighed 195 pounds and wore a size 22 dress. She had suffered from migraines, fatigue and depression for over 10 years. "I had begun to think that I would have to simply learn to adjust to this way of life," she wrote. Some way of life!

Her husband was also accommodating himself to having a wife who was overweight, always tired and depressed. Then she heard about the Bloodprint on a radio program. She took the test, and stopped eating foods to which she showed toxic reactions.

"After eight months of simply watching what I eat I now wear size 14, but I am still 39 (some things are not food related)," Dorothy wrote. "It is interesting to note that I am not particularly cutting back on the amount that I eat. I notice that when I get a headache or lack energy I can almost always trace the reaction to 'cheating' on a particular food."

Like Dorothy, Urja and thousands of others, people around the world are learning this simple fact: the right food is your first and best medicine.

"It is interesting to note that I am not particularly cutting back on the amount that I eat."

Arthritis

Arthritic sufferers have lost faith in conventional remedies and their pain is costly:

- 66% tried alternatives
- 45 million lost work days
- 39 million physician visits
- 1992 costs = $65 billion
- 60 million arthritics by 2020*

Arthritis and old age just seem to go hand-in-hand. Those joint aches and pains are "just part of growing older." Or are they?

Arthritis is actually several diseases, all of which have the same basic symptom of joint pain. Osteoarthritis is a chronic degenerative disease of the large weight-bearing joints, which comes on with age, overweight, general wear and tear, and is made worse by a lifetime of inadequate diet and exercise. Gouty arthritis is an inflammation of the joints caused by the deposition of uric acid crystals in the soft tissue of joints.

The third, and most devastating, form of arthritis is rheumatoid. This is associated with crippling disabilities, painful, tender, stiff, swollen and often deformed joints, fatigue, loss of appetite and weight, aching muscles and even anemia. Rheumatoid arthritis is classified as an

* Centers for Disease Control data reported by Houston Business Journal, Oct 29, 1999

autoimmune disease in which, doctors believe, your body mistakenly attacks its own tissues.

Osteoarthritis is, frankly, often the result of the aging process—and bad nutritional decisions made earlier in life. Gouty arthritis often responds to diet and, in some cases, medication. It is rheumatoid arthritis that is clearly linked to Toxic Food Syndrome.

Rheumatoid arthritis had silenced the music of one piano player. For 10 years, she could only look at a piano and remember when her agile hand had delighted her friends and family as they ran across the keyboard. Even heavy doses of painkillers did nothing but block the symptoms.

Then an Immuno I Bloodprint™ identified the toxic foods in her life. "The results were dramatic," she said. "In less than two days, my hands were improved. I almost cried when I realized that I might be able to play the piano again—all I had hoped for was relief from the horrors of constant pain."

"In less than two days, my hands were improved. I almost cried when I realized that I might be able to play the piano again—all I had hoped for was relief from the horrors of constant pain."

James Coburn is a world-famous actor who had a terrible family legacy: a history of hereditary rheumatoid arthritis. For years, the disease avoided him. Then it hit, and soon he was almost unable to walk or stand up without help. When a test identified the toxic foods affecting him, and he quit them, Coburn quickly improved and remained pain-free for years.

Arthritis can strike at any age. Melaney Garcia was 37 years old when she went in for some dental work. Soon after, she developed arthritic symptoms in several joints. Over the next year, her condition grew worse and worse, and she seemed to face a future of pain and immobility. That is a horrible thought when you're a mother of three very active young children.

When Melaney took her Bloodprint test, "it came back that I was sensitive to eggs and dairy," she wrote. "I took these foods out of my diet and within three days 80 percent of my pain was gone. That was three months ago. I am off all prescription and natural drugs except for Glucosamine/Chondoritin and have almost no pain." Now here's the real bottom line: "I can play basketball and baseball with my kids again and am thankful every day that I jump out of bed for that simple test that gave me my life back."

Do you see yourself in these testimonials? Is arthritis or some other disease taking your life away, either at once or bit by bit? Then you need to use nature's first and best medicine: the food you eat.

Asthma

"I begged God just to take me home."

It's no secret: there is an asthma epidemic in the world today. More and more people, from infants to seniors, are finding being able to breathe their greatest health challenge.

Take the case of Serenity Dale. "When I started, I came as a very sick, very upset lady. I have had severe allergies and asthma for about 20 years." The year before she took a blood test, "I spent the whole summer, from May 1995 through January 1996, on antibiotics and prednisone. I felt horrid. My eyes and skin were dark colored. I was having to take breathing treatments every three to four hours around the clock. I wanted to sleep. I was cranky, no energy, and I really didn't want to do anything or be around anyone. I did a lot of soul searching during that time. I begged God just to take me home. My family really was very concerned. I was sick and tired of being sick and tired."

Then, she had an Immuno 1 Bloodprint™, and eliminated the toxic foods from her life. In September 1996, she wrote, "I feel so much better and my skin isn't yucky any more. I have been able to do things I enjoy doing. We rode bikes about 14 miles a couple of weeks ago. I wasn't sure I'd ever be able to do that again. Thanks to God and your program"!

If you have asthma, or severe allergies, the real culprit may very well not be in the air you breathe, but in the food you eat. Before you condemn yourself to a life of heavy-duty medicine, try the best and first medicine: food.

Digestive Disorders

If you think toxic food seems a natural cause for digestive disorders, you're right.

But we're not talking just about indigestion or a little heartburn. Toxic foods can cause life-threatening digestive disorders, like celiac disease and Crohn's Disease.

Dr. Anahid Berberian, M.D., is a family physician and bariatrician. For 10 years, she suffered from constant heartburn, abdominal distention and diarrhea. Add to that migraine headaches, itchy skin, insomnia, a lack of energy, and palpitations.

Dr. Berberian learned about the Immuno 1 Bloodprint™ at the annual conference of the American Society of Bariatric Physicians. "It made so much sense," she wrote later, "after all, we are what we eat."

The test showed she was allergic to 15 different foods. "The result was spectacular, in three weeks my symptoms disappeared, I stopped all my medications," she wrote. "I was back being the healthy, energetic woman that I was—plus I could help all my other patients with similar symptoms."

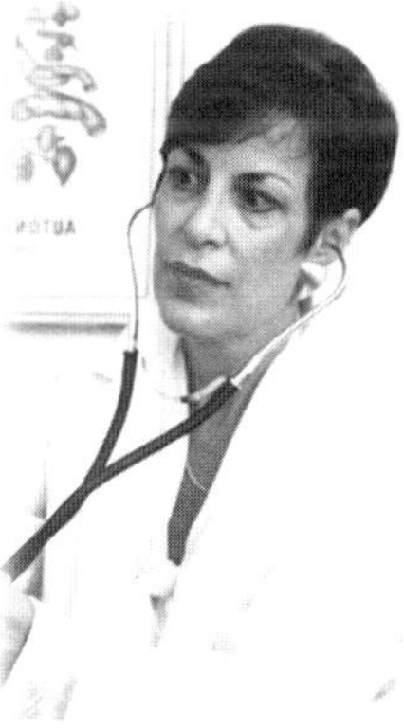

"The result was spectacular, in three weeks my symptoms disappeared, I stopped all my medications."

Another medical professional whose life was improved by the Bloodprint was Lisa Hughes, R.N., B.S.N. "I no longer have to take my daily prescription laxative," she wrote after eliminating toxic foods from her diet. "In fact, I haven't had to take a laxative for weeks! That is a miracle in itself! My pain has improved a great deal also, and my bloating is all but relieved."

"Through the years, I have suffered with spastic colitis, Irritable Bowel Syndrome, hiatal hernia, upset stomach, and [was] unable to tolerate many foods," wrote Lynn Douglas. Then her daughter introduced her to toxic food testing and the Immuno I Bloodprint™. Within weeks of changing her diet to eliminate toxic foods, her symptoms began to disappear and her health became better than any time in her life.

It is all too easy to try and make an uneasy peace with digestive problems. There are literally hundreds of over-the-counter conventional and alternative treatments out there to try and make your digestive tract work properly. All have one thing in common: they treat symptoms, not the underlying cause.

Another thing people do is limit their diet in hopes of controlling their digestive problems. But some of the blandest foods out there can be the most toxic. Dairy products often head the list of toxic foods when we test people. So is it any wonder you can't sleep after you have a glass of warm milk before going to bed to "settle your stomach?"

There's a saying in the computer business: garbage in, garbage out (that's GIGO for short). That is absolutely true when it comes to our precious digestive system: put in the garbage of an everyday food causing toxic reactions in your system, and get the garbage of bad digestion out.

Weight Loss

"I have currently lost 115 pounds."

Obesity is an absolute worldwide epidemic. Millions of us carry extra pounds that damage our health, limit our activities and shorten our lives—while sabotaging the very quality of those lives.

Sam Solomon says he ought to have known better. A hotel food and beverage director, he was trained in the proper presentation of food and drinks and also nutrition. Nevertheless, Sam tipped the scales at 365 pounds. He craved food constantly. Then he found out that he was putting toxic foods in his system. Sam changed his diet—and his life.

"At present I work the program daily," he wrote, "and although I have not met my goal weight of 180 pounds, I have currently lost 115 pounds. However, the weight loss is secondary. The most important factors are that by bringing my eating habits under control I have taken away the unhealthy tricks that food was playing on me. For example, the cravings and mood swings caused by the interaction of sugar and yeast are gone. The guilt that comes after food binges is gone. The lack of self-esteem that comes from splitting the seams of clothes, buying clothes at the fat shop or worse, and avoiding activities because one was just too big, all are gone." The bottom line, Sam told us: "I have learned to like and love myself as I was never able to do."

Janet Younger knows how crippling being overweight can be. "Before I started the elimination program, I could only stay on my feet a few minutes at a time," she wrote. "I wasn't able to shop, clean house, etc., because the pain in my ankles was too intense." After a Bloodprint and following the diet, here's what happened: "By the end of the second week I started walking for exercise," Janet said. She quickly went "from half to a full mile of walking. I can have hope for the future now."

Do you have hope for the future? Or is tomorrow just another day to try and make it through long hours of pain, discomfort, even immobility? You already know the answer to a weight problem lies in the food you eat—but perhaps you are not asking the right questions. The question, I believe, is not "How much am I eating?" but "Is the food I am eating toxic to me?" The odds are overwhelming that your eating one or more foods causing toxic reactions to your particular system if you are overweight. Throw away the diet pills and forget the latest fad diet. Just stop poisoning yourself with toxic food reactions. Turn food from your enemy to your best friend—to your first and best medicine. Relief is very likely just one simple test away.

What If You Already Feel Good?

Maybe you're reading these testimonials and thinking, "Wow, these folks have it rough. I'm glad I'm not like that!" That is exactly what one 44-year-old business executive thought. He was delighted when the Immuno I Bloodprint™ helped his children's chronic conditions, but he never imagined it would change his life.

"When I saw the test results on my children, who were both cured of conditions that medicines had failed to help (one cured of migraines and one cured of stomach aches), I decided to take the test myself," he told us. "I didn't really have any direct symptoms to speak of (at least I didn't think I did), but was curious to see if I was eating any foods that were toxic to my immune system."

So he took the test, and waited for the results—and got the surprise of his life. "I was shocked to see I had 24 food toxicities, an uncommonly high amount," he said. In fact, he had more food toxicities than his children, even though he thought (and that's the key word) he had no chronic conditions. He was about to begin a journey of self discovery.

"I removed them from my diet, lost 3 pounds the first week and feel 20 years younger," this executive said. "I simply cannot believe the difference in everything from my sex drive to my tripled daily energy, to even a notable improvement in mental acuity."

He learned what thousands of others had found: he had made peace with his chronic conditions because he could live with them (at least sort of live) and still function. "It turns out I had a lot of symptoms I had just learned to live with, including chronic fatigue, trouble sleeping and bags under my eyes (for 20 years) that went away completely." All from one test—and stopping eating the toxic foods that were robbing him of enjoying the best years of his life!

Aging

If there is a theme in this chapter, then it is that people who eliminate toxic foods from their diet get a new lease on life. After years of pain and suffering, they suddenly find freedom, new energy and, above all, hope. It's hard to have hope if your digestive tract always hurts, or if you live on antibiotics to combat sinus and ear infections, or if you are severely overweight. Now you can bring an end to merry-go-round of one more doctor, one more medicine, one more treatment—and then one more disappointment.

As we've seen, for many people hope begins when people learn many of their illnesses are a direct result of eating foods toxic to their particular system. Eliminate them, and good health comes in a matter of days.

Aging is a natural part of human life. We all age constantly, and, ultimately, we cannot stop the process. But there is a big difference between an old age of rocking chairs and fading memories, and the stories of septuagenarian marathon runners and triathletes we've already met. I don't know what their diets are like, but it is highly unlikely that they are eating foods toxic to their systems. If they were, they would have traded their running shorts for canes or walkers long ago.

You have the power to decide your future. You can go along like you are today, letting various illnesses and

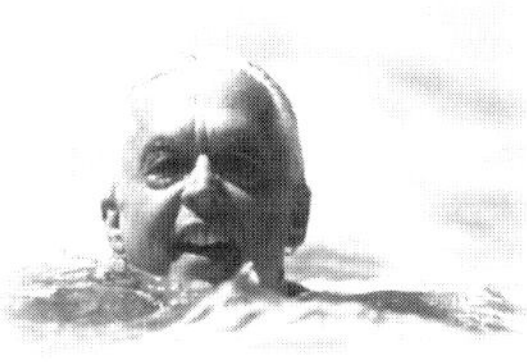

conditions, including obesity, eat you alive, bit by bit. One year, you find you can't walk a mile any more. Then comes another year, and dancing is a little too much for you. Still another year rolls along, and that television and remote control have a new prisoner. Bit by bit, your life erodes from what you once enjoyed to a mere shadow.

But you have the power to choose. Armed with the information a Bloodprint can provide, you can give up those toxic foods and shed the impact of years.

Stop making excuses like "I'm just getting older" or "What do you expect at my age?" I expect at 75 you can run a marathon—if you make the lifestyle changes you need to now. I expect at 75 you can do anything you want, if only you will stop feeding your body poison. Removing the impact of Toxic Food Syndrome is the nearest thing we have to a Fountain of Youth or a time machine. Why put up with it one day longer?

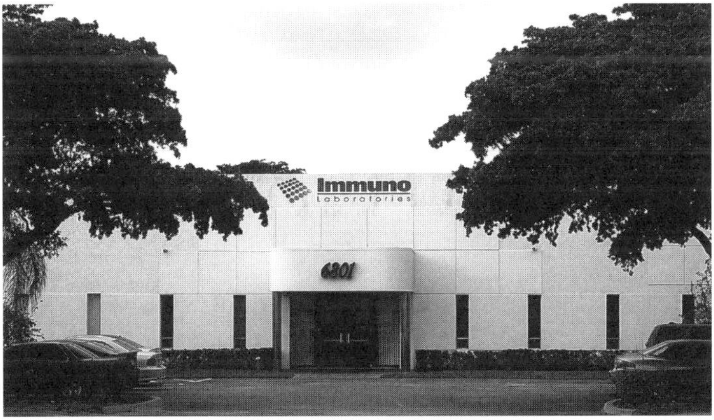

Immuno Laboratories, 6801 Powerline Road, Fort lauderdale, Florida

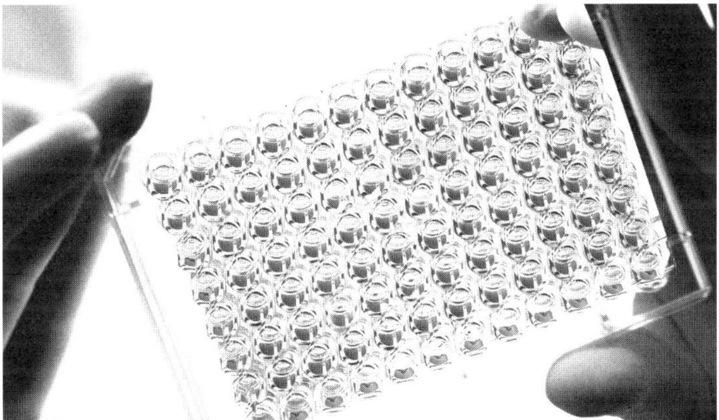

Micro titer plate—a key to precise testing and reliable test results. Immuno has invested over 15 years in the development of technology associated with the molecular amount of foods bound to each well of these plates and the multi-step process of testing your serum for toxic reactions.

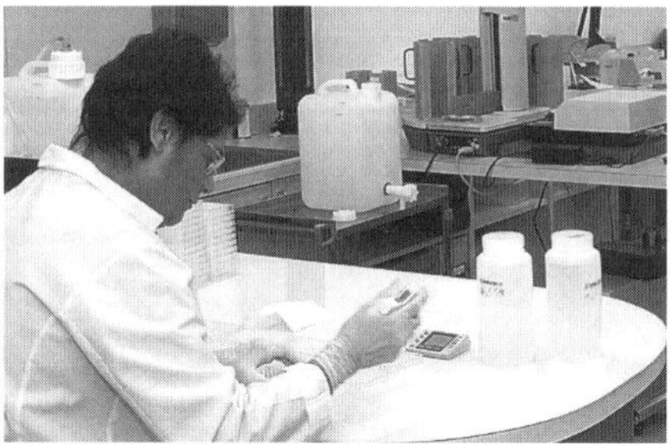

State-of-the-art facilities includes proprietary software and test procedures to ensure the most accurate and reliable test results in the world.

Automation provides the laboratory personnel with a combination of precision and efficiency as each test plate is processed. Immuno leads the way in the use of robotic and computer technology all resulting in clinically useful test results for you.

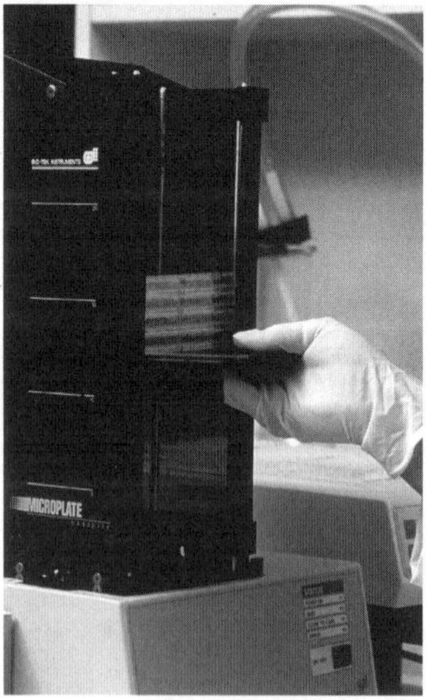

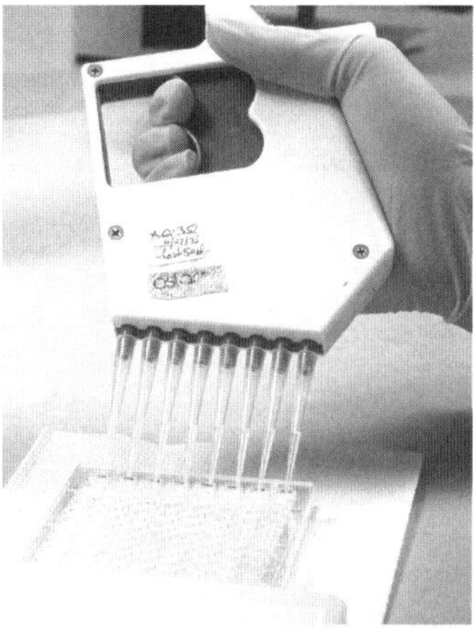

This multi-purpose instrument provides both precision and speed when it comes to dispensing precise measured amounts of your serum into the test wells. Each step in the process of testing has quality control and advanced technology to continuously produce accurate, reliable results.

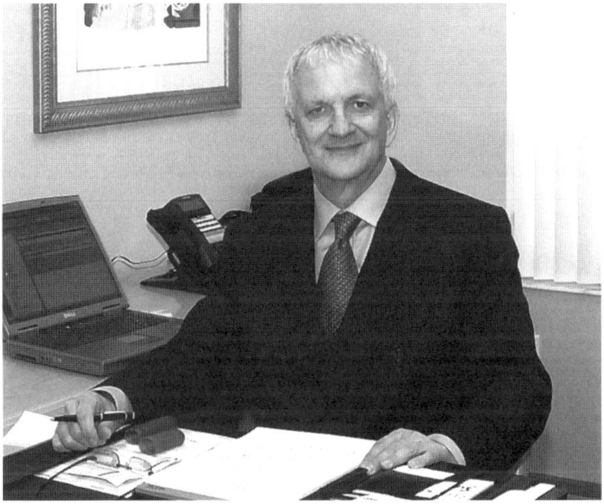

Jeffrey S. Zavik, founder and CEO, at his office in Fort Lauderdale.

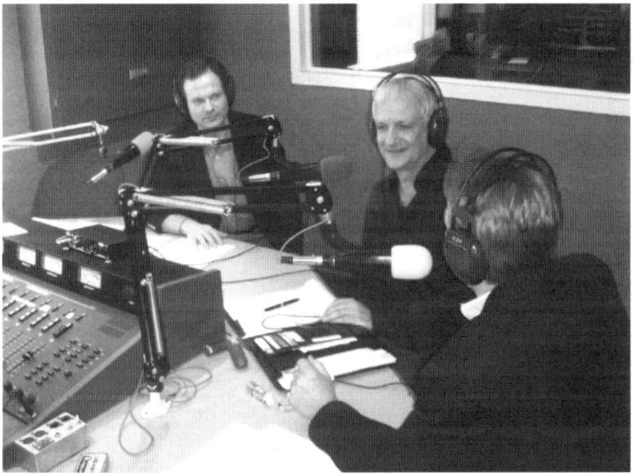

Robert Chesney, radio producer, in the studio with Dr. Louis B. Cady and author Jeffrey Zavik.

Chapter 3

How are you poisoning your body?

If you are like 95 percent of the population, you may be slowly poisoning your body every day and not even know it.

That is the sad truth about Toxic Food Syndrome. Fast-acting poisons like arsenic may take a few minutes to kill their victims, while the poison of toxic food can subject its victims to decades of living death. What else would you call a life of constant pain, respiratory problems, digestive ailments, or fatigue?

There are two kinds of toxic reactions to food. The first, called Type One, is described as immediate-onset. In other words, the victim soon knows they have eaten the wrong thing. Type One reactions take place any time within a few minutes to two hours.

Remember that scene from "Mrs. Doubtfire" I mentioned in the introduction? When Pierce Brosnan's character ate pepper, he began to choke to death. That is a Type One reaction, albeit an extreme one.

Type One reactions usually strike the skin, airway, and/or digestive tract. A rash may break out. Breathing may become difficult. Severe heartburn or other gastric distress may take place. Aside from the digestive tract, the reactions are pretty similar to what happens to someone who has a toxic reaction to something like bee venom.

While these outward symptoms take place, inside, your body is fighting what it considers a hostile invader. We all learned back in high school biology how antibodies appear in the bloodstream to attack bacteria and toxic substances in our bloodstream. When you have a Type One toxic reaction to food, your body interprets the food as an "enemy" and attacks it with antibodies. Cells called "mast cells" produce histamines, which can inhibit your ability to breathe. Did you ever wonder why anti-allergy medicines are called "antihistamines"? They control your allergy symptoms by clearing up histamines. The result is a virtual battle in your body, and the symptoms you experience are the byproduct.

So you eat and start sneezing or notice your nose is running. That's the "good" end of the Type One reaction scale. The "bad" extreme to Type One is fortunately uncommon—a fatal reaction to a food. That is called anaphylaxis, which can cause the rapid swelling of a person's tongue and throat, and even a drop in blood pressure and an irregular heart beat.

Type One toxic reactions are usually pretty easy to identify. By the third or fourth time you've had, let's say, shellfish, and felt sick immediately afterwards, you'll get the picture a particular food is not for you. If the reaction is severe enough, the problem will likely be diagnosed by a medical doctor—possibly in an emergency room.

Then there is a second type of toxic reaction. These Type Two reactions are called "delayed onset." The name is self-explanatory: Type Two toxic reactions to food may take as long as three days to appear.

What happens is the body reacts slower in these cases to the toxic food. Often, the symptoms are similar to Type One, but they are often less severe. No one, for example, would have their windpipe almost close from something they ate three days earlier. But there are many symptoms which can occur, as we've seen. In chapter 6, there is a checklist of symptoms which can occur from Type Two toxic reactions. There is an amazing variety of symptoms, as you can see from this list.

Type One reactions are relatively easy to spot. But that is not the case with Type Two toxic reactions, and the reason is time.

Imagine the variety of foods you eat in 72 hours—three whole days. At the end of that time, you have symptoms. But which food caused it? And was it a "complete" food, like an ear of corn, or was it a pre-packaged food with a seasoning or spice hidden way far down in the contents label?

Try this. Write down everything you eat for one day. Not just the main courses, but add in all the different items contained in the food you eat. You will be amazed by what you find, and how many ingredients are actually in the food you consume. And any one or more of them may be poisoning you. **So now what do you do?**

Summary Chart

Immediate reaction

1. Only one or two (rarely more) foods involved in causing toxic symptoms.
2. Small, even trace amounts of food can trigger an intense allergic reaction.
3. Toxic symptoms commonly appear two hours or less after consuming offending foods.
4. Primarily affects the skin, airway and digestive tract.
5. Common in children, rare in adults.
6. Addictive cravings and withdrawal symptoms are rare to non-existent.
7. With the exception of infants and young children, the toxic food is often self-diagnosed. This is because only one or two foods are usually involved, and the onset of toxic symptoms occurs quickly.
8. Type One food reactions occur with foods you eat infrequently.
9. Commonly a permanent, fixed food allergy.
10. Frequently produces a positive result to conventional skin testing for food allergies.

Delayed reaction

1. Three to ten toxic foods may be involved, though 20 or more are found in some cases. Rare for only one or two foods to be toxic this way.
2. Larger amounts of food, often in multiple feedings, commonly needed to produce toxic symptoms. Reactions may not occur from a single helping of food.
3. Allergic symptoms commonly appear 2 to 24 hours after toxic foods are eaten. Symptoms appearing 48 to 72 hours later have been reported.
4. Virtually any tissue, organ, or system of the body can be affected.
5. Very common in children and adults. Well over 50 medical conditions and 200 symptoms have been reported to be provoked, worsened or caused by toxic reactions to foods.
6. Addictive cravings and withdrawal symptoms clinically significant in 20 to 30 percent of patients.
7. Due to the number of foods involved and the delayed onset of symptoms, successful self-diagnosis is rare. Multiple doctor visits involving different physicians are the rule, not the exception, before proper diagnosis and treatment is provided.
8. Toxic foods are commonly favorite foods, frequently eaten, and eaten in larger amounts.
9. Toxic reactions to foods are commonly reversible. Symptoms often clear after three to six months of avoidance and nutritional therapy.
10. Skin tests for allergic reactions to these foods are negative.

Chapter 4

How to test yourself for food toxicities

If you are unfortunate enough to have a Type One toxic reaction to food, it is often fairly simple for a physician to determine the cause. If the reaction is mild enough, some people will attempt to solve the puzzle themselves, by simple trial and error. Eat this, don't eat that and see what happens.

It is also possible to do self-testing with Type Two toxic reactions. Most people will eliminate a whole group of foods, such as dairy or grain products, and see if their health improves.

The problem is the delay in reaction, and the complexity of the food we eat. You can't very well eat something, not eat again for three days and see if you have a reaction! That sounds ridiculous, but that is exactly what it would take to determine your Type Two toxic reactions to food by the trial and error method.

Fortunately, there is an answer, which is simple, relatively painless, effective and reasonably priced. That is an Immuno I Bloodprint™. Here is how it works: You start with a licensed phlebotomist (someone trained to draw your blood) usually right in your doctor's office. At times, we will assist your doctor in arranging to have your blood draw done in your home or office by appointment. Sterile, disposable supplies are used and all the preparation and shipping of your sample is handled.

Having a sample of blood drawn is all you have to do to have the Immuno 1 Bloodprint™ test completed. At the lab, highly trained technicians inject a small sample of your blood into tiny micro titer plate wells. These look like glass contact lenses. These wells contain 115 different food antigens. These antigens have been optimized by a proprietary method developed by Dr. John Rebello, the scientist who perfected this test and oversees all such testing.

How the test works:

Step 1

Lab techs inject a sampling of your serum into micro titer wells coated with 115 different food antigens.

Step 2

Over a few hours, antibodies in your serum interact with the food antigens (optimized by the Rebello method); enzyme conjugate is then added which binds to specific antibody. Next, enzyme substrate is added and within minutes a visible color change occurs in each well containing the specific allergic antibody.

Step 3

A high tech scanner with laser-like beams of light reads and records the toxic reactions your serum has as it interfaces with each food. State-of-the-art computers report the reactions in 4 categories of reactivity.

The information gathered by this highly sophisticated micro plate scanner is then processed through special laboratory computers. These quantify the reactions to each of 115 antigens and rank them within four categories.

Notice that none of this is subjective. The lab technicians do not decide whether there is a reaction or how strong it is. All that is handled by electronic equipment, specially designed for this purpose.

While the process is sophisticated, the test result you will receive is clear, concise and easy to read and understand. Your report will include:

- A list of toxic foods to avoid
- A list of foods (lots of them!) to enjoy
- A wallet-sized, laminated reminder card listing your particular toxic foods
- Your personalized food and meal plan
- Helpful hints for food shopping

Reliable Testing

There are several laboratories out there that perform blood testing to determine food toxicities. It is critical to know, however, that you are working with a quality lab to insure accurate test results.

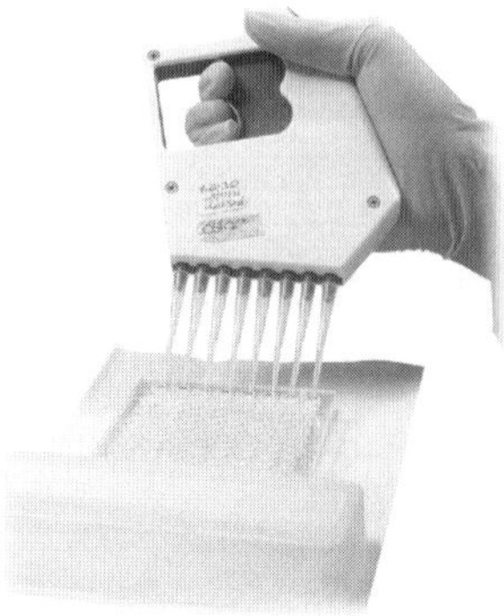

Frankly, you can't have a good lab without a good director. Dr. Jeffrey Bland, CEO of HealthComm Inc. and former professor of chemistry of the University of Puget Sound, director of the Bellevue-Redmond Medical Laboratory, and research associate at the Linus Pauling Laboratory for Nutrient Analysis, said, "I believe Dr. John Rebello is one of the best, if not the best, laboratory directors I've met." I agree entirely.

"I believe Dr. John Rebello is one of the best, if not the best, laboratory directors I've met."

But let me allow Dr. Rebello to tell his own story: "Let me go back to Bombay, India, where I was raised and where I received my early, more basic education. In Bombay, I'm what you might call the product of a very solid Jesuit Catholic education.

"By the time I attended high school, my interests were already in science. I entered St. Xavier's College in Bombay,

India, where I graduated with honors with a major in microbiology and a minor in chemistry. Immediately after graduation I applied for graduate school at the same college and had the very good fortune of receiving a 'demonstratorship' in the microbiology department, which is equivalent to a teaching assistantship here in America."

Dr. Rebello earned his master's degree in microbiology. "My master's thesis was 'Anti-viral Principles from Indian Medicinal Plants.' After I finished my teaching assistantship, I was given an assistant professorship at St. Xavier's."

In the early 1960s, Dr. Rebello moved to the United States to continue his education. "I started my doctoral program in the department of biochemistry at the State University of New York in Buffalo, in August 1964." There, he worked with Dr. Norman Strauss, an internationally recognized expert in branch-point enzymes. In 1968, after completing his doctorate, Dr. Rebello received a special fellowship to work with Dr. Roy Jensen in the department of microbiology and immunology at the Baylor College of Medicine in Houston.

After two years at Baylor, Dr. Rebello accepted another teaching and research position, this one at Texas A & M University, in their department of biochemistry. He also worked for biomedical companies in Houston and Miami and his work focused on human plasma proteins, generating assays for specific immunoglobulins. Dr. Rebello trained with Kari Cantell, M.D., PhD, the father of interferon research, and continued work on interferon and early development of HIV testing.

Then, in August 1986, he joined Immuno Laboratories as its director. Today, he is still at that post, assuring our high quality testing and results.

"I strongly believe that a good laboratory begins with a well-trained staff of technicians and technologists," Dr. Rebello says. "It's the director who must make sure that the laboratory possesses all current equipment, reagents and testing procedures so that well trained technicians can perform the accurate, reproducible assays every time, day in and day out."

If I may interject into Dr. Rebello's comments, "reproducible" is a critical word in any testing. If you were a woman, you wouldn't want to have a pregnancy test that one time said you were going to have a baby—and the next time said you would not. Imagine if the results of a test for cancer varied and gave false positives. So one of Dr. Rebello's main goals—and accomplishments—is to make sure Immuno's blood tests produce the same results for one individual every time.

There is a dark secret in the blood testing industry. There are simply too many labs out there that cannot produce consistent, reproducible test results. Some people have tested this, sending split samples from the same person—and getting different results from each. You might as well flip a coin to decide which foods are toxic for you.

Dr. Rebello developed Immuno's stringent, three-level quality control program. Because of his international experience in his field, he would accept nothing but a process that would meet the highest standards of his profession. That includes an unannounced split sample test sent through the technicians at least weekly. "Every week I select a patient's serum with a known amount of positives in it," Dr. Rebello says. "I then split this sample for duplicate testing. I anticipate and demand that this particular split will give me the same number and kind of positive and negative foods in both runs."

I feel honored to be associated with John Rebello. Here is a man who has spent his life working to improve the lives of others, first in a variety of biochemical research, then in the battle against cancer and AIDS, and now in helping millions conquer the true source of their problems: toxic food. To each field, he has brought his great knowledge and skills, as well as his commitment to quality and scientific accuracy. Thanks to him and his staff, Immuno Laboratories is your best choice for blood tests for food toxicity in the world.

Chapter 5

Remember my story?

Toxic Food Syndrome has plagued most of my life and the story continues to this present day. With all that I've learned, I've been able to enjoy incredibly better health and minimum symptoms by eliminating foods toxic to my particular system. But, a new twist of events produced yet another important insight for me. In 1998, I periodically had bouts of pain in my stomach area. I was already eating the right foods, exercising regularly and the pain puzzled me. I slipped back into the symptom treatment type of mindset and began numbing the pain with aspirin. I did this as needed for several years, ignoring what my body might be telling me. Then, in 2000, the pain worsened and the aspirin ceased to kill the pain. I sought medical advice and the first doctor's conclusion was "it's your gallbladder." I ended up in the hospital for ultra sound and then a CAT scan, which included a special intravenous dye to help the doctors assess my condition. I was pretty scared. As it turned out, they found absolutely nothing wrong and I was relieved from my fears of cancer and other crazy worries, but still left with my pain. My doctor still felt it would be best to remove the gallbladder. I decided to remove the doctor instead and sought a new doctor that might offer better advice. I feel very fortunate because my new physician gave my symptoms more careful consideration. He asked me lots of good questions all about my symptoms and looked somewhat puzzled. On one hand, the diagnosis seemed like it involved my gallbladder but high tech testing did not support such a diagnosis. He told me the only other likely explanation would be an ulcer. I immediately disagreed—couldn't imagine I'd have an ulcer. But, to make a long story short, the aspirin I used to kill my pain probably created an ulcer. It all made sense! I was so puzzled why low fat, fresh foods eaten in a Japanese restaurant would produce intense pain—answer: I loved the spicy horseradish seasoning called wasabi and generously used it on my Japanese meal. I also wondered why Indian food produced extreme tiredness and headaches. Of course, the food was very spicy. And, last of all my unanswered questions was waking up without having eaten anything at all with incredible pain—the stomach acids through the night were irritating the ulcer.

The right food is your first and best medicine and the right doctor will see to it that any other factors affecting your health will be properly treated and cared for.

The lesson learned here is the importance of forging a partnership with the right doctor. The right food is your first and best medicine and the right doctor will see to it that any other factors affecting your health will be properly treated and cared for. I highly recommend seeking such a physician. One cautionary note to you: there are imitators out there who'll have you testing your blood and offering it as the total cure for everything that ails you. While I agree that Toxic Food Syndrome is rampant and it's very important to identify and eliminate foods that are toxic for you—still your health and well being involve more than just the food you eat. Please don't ignore this fact and find yourself a doctor with whom you can build a trusting, cooperative relationship. The right doctor will assist you and support you; the right doctor will honor and respect your desire to participate in the choices that you make for your healthcare. And, the right doctor will also be open to the idea that the right food is your first and best medicine. Take your test through your doctor and add a safety net to your lifetime of optimal health.

The great news about toxic food testing is how simple it really is. You take your test and receive your test results. Your program primarily consists of the following: food avoidance, food rotation, food diary, tracking your progress with your symptom checklist and reintroducing the foods you avoided. Your partnership with the right doctor will assist you with your toxic food testing program. Your doctor will assist you in 3 or more important ways: having your blood professionally and painlessly drawn for the test; assessing your symptoms and checking you thoroughly to be certain other contributing factors to your overall health are properly addressed, tested and treated as is necessary, and providing ongoing support as you proceed on your toxic food elimination program.

Chapter 6

Do You Suffer From Toxic Food Syndrome?

Attention, everybody: it's time for a test.

In the next few minutes, you will take one of the most important tests of your life. By the time you are done, you will know if you, like 95 percent of all people, suffer from Toxic Food Syndrome.

If you do, then the symptoms you see here may not have to be part of your life. I'm serious. You may be just weeks away from leaving these conditions behind forever. That is what makes this test so important. Years from now, you may well look back at this as the first step you took to taking back your life. One last note: if you are a parent, you can take this test for your child, or help your child complete it. Now let's begin: Use this point scale to rate your symptoms based on how you've been feeling during the past 30 days:

0 = Never or almost never had the symptom
1 = Occasionally had it, but the effect was not severe
2 = Occasionally had it, and the effect was severe
3 = Frequently had it, but the effect was not severe
4 = Frequently had it, and the effect was severe

Let's look at those numbers. If you scored 3 or 4 on any one symptom or your total score is above 10 in any one category or your total score is greater than 50, the odds are high you suffer from Toxic Food Syndrome. If it seemed like the Symptom checklist test read almost like the story of your health, there is every chance the food you eat is standing between you and the health you desire so desperately. Fortunately, while some food causes toxic reactions for you, food itself remains your first and best medicine in the quest for good health.

Now it is time for some self-examination. Looking back at your scores on the symptom checklist, do you see how a variety of symptoms you may have dismissed have accumulated? What has happened to you, as to so many people—myself included—is you have tried to make peace with your ailments. You don't want to be one of those people who only talk about your aches and pains. So you tough it out and try to "play with pain." You adjust your lifestyle not to match the desires of you or your family, but the demands of your illnesses and disabilities.

Not too far from where I wrote this book in western North Carolina is the home of a truly remarkable man. Millions around the world have enjoyed the brilliant guitar playing of Doc Watson. Many know he has been blind almost his entire life. Instead of "making peace" with that fact, Doc has lived life to its fullest, performing around the world, raising a family, and inventing a style of guitar playing admired everywhere.

The roots of his success lie in his childhood. His father, General Dixon Watson, would not let his son just be a "poor blind boy." As soon as the child was able, the father put him on one end of a two-man crosscut saw in the woods. He instilled independence in the boy, and a feeling of accomplishment and self-worth. Even in recent years, Doc has been known to climb up and help men fixing the roof on his house.

Even facing such a disability as blindness, Doc Watson and many others have carved out successful lives, and refused to surrender to their challenges. That is the attitude you need today, if you have allowed your "aches and pains" to take over your life.

Play back the last few weeks. Do sentences like this come to mind? "Bill, I'd love to play a round of golf, but this knee of mine..." Or "I wish I could watch the grandchildren, but I just can't keep up with them." Or "Sorry, son, but I'm just worn out."

That last sentence makes me think back to a hit song of my generation, "Cat's in the Cradle" by Harry Chapin. If you say things like "Sorry, kids, I'm beat" all the time, you need to listen to this song and think about really hard. Your kids will grow up all too fast. Are you able to enjoy their youth with them?

If that has made you feel a little uncomfortable, here is something else to think about. If you, like me, are "middle aged," you may be putting off your symptoms as part of the aging process. "I just can't go like I used to." "My get up and go has got up and went." "What do you expect when you get to be ..."

As we saw back in the introduction, what some people expect to do when they pass the 75 year mark is run marathons and complete triathlons! Why are you willing to accept less—at least without a fight?

I had a dear friend many years ago who started aging himself out of activities while he was still in his 40's. First, he started to cut back on outdoor excursions and hikes. Soon, he spent more and more time at home, living quietly. It wasn't long before he was an old man—and not just chronologically. What a waste!

Take a hard look at your symptoms—and declare war on them. The place to start is to identify your enemies—with a blood test. When you know and avoid the foods toxic to your particular system, you will soon be able to claim victory over your symptoms, just like the people we featured in Chapter 2. Today is the day to get on the road to a new life.

Take a hard look at your symptoms—and declare war on them.

Chapter 7

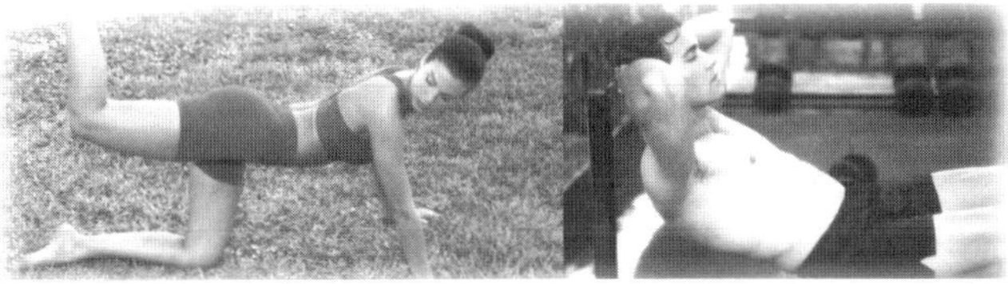

The Right Food Is Your First And Best Medicine

I won't lay claim to inventing the idea that the right food is your best medicine, but my crusade elevates this truth to a whole new level. Not only is the right food your best medicine, it's your ***first*** and best medicine. Before doing anything more drastic or costly, FIRST be certain you are fueling your body properly by eating the foods that are right for your particular system.

Before doing anything more drastic or costly, FIRST be certain you are fueling your body properly by eating the foods that are right for your particular system.

People have known for thousands of years that food and health are intimately connected. Even before any had thought of what we call the scientific method, Greeks and Romans had figured out "we are what we eat."

The Roman philosopher Lucretius, in his book "De Rerum Natura" (On Natural Things), wrote "What is food to one, is to others bitter poison." Isn't that amazing? Two thousand years ago, without even the simplest scientific tools, Lucretius understood this fundamental truth. What that tells me is the link between health and food is obvious. There is no mystery: you can figure it out by looking at the people around you.

The first medical doctor of ancient times, at least in the West, was the Greek, Hippocrates. Even today, new physicians take the Hippocratic Oath, which defines the nature and ethics of their profession. In his book "Precepts," Hippocrates wrote: "Healing is a matter of time, but it is sometimes also a matter of opportunity." That is another great truth: sometimes our bodies require time to heal, but other times there comes an opportunity to made a rapid gain in health. Conquering Toxic Food Syndrome with this blood test is such an opportunity.

These ancients were wise in other ways. Hippocrates (in "Regimen in Health") also wrote, "A wise man should consider that health is the greatest of human blessings, and learn how by his own thought to derive benefit from his illnesses."

Think about that for a minute. There is no question health is the "greatest of human blessings," but most of us think sickness is the "greatest of human curses." Hippocrates would not have agreed, because he was wise enough to realize that illnesses are our body's way of warning us something is wrong.

I have known a number of people who suffered mild heart attacks, adopted a healthier lifestyle and enjoyed years of good health. Many others have had a variety of symptoms, consulted a medical professional and found their "curse" was in fact a timely warning.

If you have some or even many of the symptoms outlined in Chapter 6, you can "derive benefit from" your illnesses. If you are suffering from Toxic Food Syndrome, your body's symptoms are trying to tell you something: help, I'm being poisoned! Are you ready to listen and are you ready to do something about it?

"A wise man should consider that health is the greatest of human blessings, and learn how by his own thought to derive benefit from his illnesses."

Right now, you may be someone who has suffered a variety of symptoms for many years, and be so discouraged that you are about ready to give up. I remember one letter, quoted in Chapter 2, from a woman who literally begged God to take her home. That is something you want to understand when you finish this book: no matter how long you have suffered, the situation is not hopeless. Don't stand at the door of success, too weary to open one more door.

Take the example of Thomas Alva Edison, the man who invented the light bulb, phonograph, motion pictures and hundreds of other inventions. Edison succeeded not because he had flashes of genius that helped him invent things, but because he never gave up. In inventing the light bulb, Edison tried over 6,000 different materials for the filament. Only the last one worked. Had he not tried that one more time, his name would be forgotten.

Edison put it this way: "I have not failed. I've just found 10,000 ways that won't work." His secret was he was always willing to try the ten thousand and first way, and the ten thousand and second way. Does that sound like your experience with trying to find medical help for your symptoms? I believe the Bloodprint is that ten thousand and first way you've been seeking.

As Edison also said, "Many of life's failures are people who did not realize how close they were to success when they gave up. "What a tragedy, to give up when success—in this case good health—is just within reach."

"Many of life's failures are people who did not realize how close they were to success when they gave up."

Edison also had something to say to those who are willing to give up their lives bit by bit by accepting the defeats illnesses, conditions and painful or annoying symptoms try to hand us. To those who adapt or put it off on aging, Edison said two things:

"Restlessness and discontent are the first necessities of progress." And "If we did all the things we are capable of, we would literally astound ourselves."

Don't accept limitations, and don't accept defeat. Get discontented with your life, seek the proper help I have outlined in this book—and then get ready to astound yourself and others with what you can do!

The bottom line here is simple: health is our greatest treasure. The wealthy invalid would trade her mansion and wealth for health and vigor. One of the wisest men of the last century, Mahatma Gandhi, put it this way: "It is health that is real wealth and not pieces of gold and silver."

Changing Times, Changing Attitudes—Times are changing, and so are attitudes.

There was a time when large disease-related organizations vehemently denied that diet and disease went hand in hand. Twenty-five or thirty years ago, groups like the American Cancer Society and the various arthritis groups looked for solutions other than the food we eat. If someone suggested an "anti-cancer" diet, conventional wisdom would reject it.

How times have changed! Just watch an old **health education** newsreel from the 1950s, and you'll see why. They have a man in a suit, explaining how we all need to regularly eat lots of red meat, cheese, and other foods. In just a little more than a generation, that version of healthy eating has gone completely out the window. Today, scientists have shown how diets heavy in fat can lead to certain forms of cancer, and how cholesterol (a word you never heard back in those days) can cause fatal heart problems. In other words, diet has a direct impact on your health.

Go visit the web sites of organizations that raise funds for research on various chronic diseases. You'll find papers and other information, all of it dealing with the connection of diet and that particular disease. Some only 'suggest' that there's a diet connection; others clearly acknowledge a diet connection. That is a huge change from the past.

At Immuno Laboratories, we are at the cutting edge of this quantum shift in how we view diet and disease. Our work follows the overall pattern of medical science, which has, historically, moved to identify problems that are more and more subtle.

The earliest physicians could only treat surface ailments; surgery was unknown. They were limited to what their eyes could see and their fingers touch.

Later, surgery was developed, and then various ways of non-intrusively looking inside the body, including X-rays, CAT and MRI scans. As each developed, smaller objects could be seen. The first glimpse of a malignant tumor now came when it was still tiny and a cure was possible. The tiniest imperfection in an organ could be detected.

That is what has happened with food. In ancient times, people would call a food poisonous—toxic—if it immediately killed someone or made them sick. Only the most obvious connections could be observed.

Later, science discovered what was called food "allergies," a very limited view and a part of which I prefer to call Toxic Food Syndrome. But all they found was the immediate reaction, something that happens involving a few certain foods over a period of a few hours.

Gradually, physicians began to notice more and more subtle reactions to food. A colleague of mine has a friend who was one of the greatest scientists in the 20th century. His research led to key breakthroughs in medical technology, and has led to the saving of many lives. A quarter century ago, however, he seemed to be near the end of his life. He developed terrible digestive problems, lost weight—he was already a thin man—and appeared to be dying. Cancer was suspected, but no one could find a trace of the disease. Finally, a wise doctor learned the truth: he was allergic to gluten! As soon as he stopped eating that toxic food, his health improved immediately and he remains a much sought-after lecturer and researcher today.

It was because of cases like that the Immuno I Bloodprint™ came into existence. Having seen the truth about what food could do to you in my own life, I wanted to save others from decades of suffering. And that is what Immuno Laboratories is all about.

The biggest change in how we think about the food-disease link has come in medical offices around the world. A generation ago, most physicians would have recommended you eat what the federal government called a healthy diet. Now we know that was a diet that could make you sick. It was not the fault of the doctors—they were going with the best information they had available.

Today, most every physician talks about a healthy diet. At the cutting edge of this trend, there are now physicians all across America and beyond our shores who are authorized providers of the Immuno 1 Bloodprint™. That itself shows the tremendous shift in the medical attitude nationally. If I had gone to doctors in the 1950s with this test, many of them would have ignored me completely. But today a growing number of medical professionals are endorsing this test and recommending it to their patients. That is the best testimony to its scientific validity.

In the future, I strongly believe we will see Toxic Food Syndrome recognized as the killer it really is. I believe it will be talked about in medical offices everywhere, and people will understand that old Lucretius was right when he wrote so many years ago, "What is food to one, is to others bitter poison."

Chapter 8

The Future of Healthcare

Why people seek alternative treatments:*

- Frustration
- Treated more humanely
- More resources from cultures worldwide
- Scientific evidence
- Wellness
- Safer
- Save money
- Increasingly supported by prominent MD's

People are once again getting involved in their own healthcare.

When medicine and science combined for the first time in the 18th century, the art of healing started to become more and more complicated and technical. By the middle of this century, many people simply followed their doctor's advice and let healthcare to the professionals.

Dissatisfaction with modern medicine began to surface in the 1960s, as part of a generation turning away from the "establishment." People began to look to herbs, Eastern practices, Native Americans and other sources to find more natural, less intrusive means of healing. Most importantly, they decided to look at people as whole beings, rather than

*American Journal of Health Promotion Nov/Dec 1997: 112-122

a series of lesser parts with separate ailments. The word "holistic" entered the English vocabulary as a way of describing this whole medicine. These natural doctors tried to find underlying causes of illness. Many recognized diet as critical to good health.

Today, the young people of the 1960s are approaching retirement age. As their bodies have aged, many have come to appreciate modern medicine more, but they have kept two important lessons from their youth.

The first of these is to be an informed, even skeptical consumer of healthcare. Many people today are unwilling just to listen and obey. The sales of medical reference works to the general public and the millions of visits annually to on-line medical web sites both speak to that. Healthcare consumers have become medical researchers, no longer willing to simply take a physician's word for it. That is a healthy trend, which is good for both consumers and doctors.

The second critical lesson they have kept is to look at their bodies as a whole. The holistic trend has spread from the grassroots, the average person, to the medical profession. Increasingly, people are not satisfied with suppressing symptoms and trying to go on. They want to find the root of the problem and solve it. That is an excellent attitude.

The result of all this is that most people today do not want a boss-employee or teacher-student relationship with their medical doctor. Instead, they want to be partners with their physician. They want to be in control of their healthcare, aware and informed.

This is particularly important because of the vast changes that have taken place in the medical field in recent decades. More than ever, healthcare has become business, not because doctors are more focused on money but because insurance companies, HMOs and other managed care organizations are so deeply involved.

Your doctor must spend more and more time on business issues to simply survive in the modern medical world. And when HMOs and Medicare, rather than the physician and patient, dictate how long someone remains in the hospital, it is clearly time to get involved.

That is what the Immuno I Bloodprint™ is all about: taking control of your life. It is about not settling for "one size fits all" nutrition advice; it is about recognizing you and your body are unique and have special needs. The Bloodprint is a critical step in determining the nature of those needs.

Think of the Bloodprint as a map of your body's nutritional needs. In reviewing your report, you will immediately learn the safe and toxic foods and, with that knowledge, map your eating to insure optimal health.

Cost

Cost is an important consideration in any healthcare program. Even though good health is priceless, we all face the reality that money does matter.

The good news about the Bloodprint is you already are spending your treatment dollars—and they are already in your budget. Following this test, your treatment consists of eliminating certain foods from your diet. You already shop for groceries and have a monthly food budget, so all you have to do is eliminate some foods and purchase more of others. The cost is likely to remain similar.

In fact, after the first few weeks, your weekly bill at the supermarket may well decline. That is definitely true if you have suffered from food cravings and binge eating. When you, like many others, find those urges are gone, you will see the amount of food you need to buy decline.

There is, of course, an upfront cost of having the test itself. Fortunately, this is well within the means of most people. If you question the cost, take a minute to think about this. Right now, if you are like 95 percent of all people, you suffer from Toxic Food Syndrome, you are spending your money to poison yourself. That's right, you are not only being poisoned—but you are paying for the "privilege"!

Let's say dairy products are toxic for you, a common result we find in testing. By the way, it's not surprising many people do have a toxic reaction to dairy products. After all, the milk most of us drink is perfectly designed to be nutritious—for calves!

Back to the point. Imagine dairy products are toxic for you. Take a few minutes and figure out how much you spend on dairy products each week. Perhaps several gallons of milk, butter, cream for your coffee, then the many items that contain dairy products. Add that all up, and you will you may be spending the cost of an Immuno I Bloodprint™ in just a few weeks—and poisoning yourself in the process.

So far, we have just talked about money. But that is only part of the picture. When someone is injured in an accident, and the other person is at fault, a court will often award damages for "pain and suffering." There is no real way to put a price tag on pain, but judges and juries try to compensate victims in such cases. If the "jury" of the Immuno I Bloodprint™ comes back and finds, let's say, wheat guilty of causing your chronic symptoms, you might have 10, 20 or 30 years of "pain and suffering" from what that toxic food has done to you. Wouldn't discovering the culprits behind your chronic problems be worth the price of one test?

There are other considerations to look at as well. How many days of work did you miss last year because of chronic conditions? How many days did you just not have the energy you would have liked at work? Did that big promotion go to someone else because of your absences and fatigue? Think about it. Besides pain and suffering, your chronic symptoms could be damaging your career.

Finally, there is one more group of bills to consider. What do your chronic symptoms cost you in medical expenses each year? How much time do you spend tracking down one more specialist, or heading off to your regular physician? Do they know you by your first name at every doctor's office in town? Are medical expenses a constant part of your items deductions? Take a few minutes and add those up.

When you put all the numbers together—food costs, pain and suffering, lost work and opportunities, and medical expenses, I think you will agree that the Immuno I Bloodprint™ test is a bargain.

There's one more thing I need to mention. Unlike almost any other medical procedure you can name, the Bloodprint comes with a money-back guarantee. Here are the six terms and conditions of our money back offer:

1) You are currently experiencing one or more of the following chronic symptoms: headaches, indigestion, overweight, fatigue, sinus congestion or arthritic pain. For your children: hyperactivity, attention deficit disorder or otitis media (ear infections).

2) Before beginning your 90-day program you complete the Initial Symptom Checklist found on page 36 of the Immuno Health Guide.

3) You maintain your Daily Food Records found following page 40 in the Immuno Health Guide for a minimum of 21 consecutive days and your journal entries document that you have avoided your toxic food list and your adherence to the Immuno Food Plan. (It's generally recognized to take a minimum of 21 days to change habits.)

4) You complete the Symptom Progress Checklist #1, #2, and #3 found on pages 37 through 39 of the Immuno Health Guide every 30 days to document your progress and turn them in to your healthcare professional as they are completed.

5) If after 90 days you have not experienced measurable improvement you may return your completed Daily Food Records, Initial Symptom Checklist, the 3 Symptom Progress Checklists of the Immuno Health Guide and your laboratory test results. Upon receipt of these items, we will refund your entire Immuno 1 Bloodprint ™ (IgG) testing fee. Your claim must be made within the first 120 days of testing. This offer is subject to change without notice.

6) This offer is not available when your testing is provided via insurance assignment.

Looking Ahead

Frankly, I'm never going to be entirely satisfied with the Immuno I Bloodprint™ – the same way Thomas Edison was not satisfied with his first light bulb. Since I started Immuno Laboratories back in 1978, I have worked with my team there to keep on the cutting edge—and beyond—of modern technology. When John Rebello joined the team in 1986, we took a quantum leap forward and haven't stopped progressing since.

In the next several years, I see the Immuno I Bloodprint™ offering deeper and deeper insights into the human body. You will be able to learn more and more about yourself and what is happening inside you through this simple test. The day will come when food toxicity will be only one of the things you will learn from your report.

Right now, we are heading toward that goal. Keep in touch with your authorized provider for exciting developments, or for the latest news, visit our website at **www.BetterHealthUSA.com**.

One final point: just because new developments are on the way is no reason to delay your testing. Back in Edison's time, people quickly adopted the first light bulbs. They didn't sit around in the darkness on the expectation something better was just around the corner. Why suffer another day? Call your doctor now and schedule your Immuno I Bloodprint™—get yourself and your loved ones on the road to better health. If you want to be referred to a physician familiar with this testing, in the USA, call toll free: 800-231-9197. All other inquiries, call 954-691-2500.

A special invitation to healthcare providers reading this book: we are very interested in expanding our qualified providers list. The inquiries for the Immuno 1 Bloodprint™, our unique method of toxic food testing is growing exponentially. In the interest of providing our consumer inquiries the best possible support, we have set standards that qualify providers. You are invited to see if your practice qualifies and if it does qualify, we'd be happy to refer people to you who are seeking toxic food testing in your area. If you are accepting new patients and meet our qualification standards, we'll welcome you aboard.

If you have one or more of these symptoms, there's a 95% probability you'll benefit from a food toxicity test.

Digestive Tract
____Diarrhea
____Constipation
____Bloated feeling
____Belching
____Passing gas
____Stomach pains

Ears
____Itchy ears
____Ear aches
____Ear infections
____Drainage from ear
____Ringing in ears
____Hearing loss

Emotions
____Mood swings
____Anxiety, fear
____Irritability, anger
____Depression
____Aggressiveness
____Nervousness

Energy & Activity
____Fatigue
____Sluggishness
____Apathy
____Hyperactivity
____Restlessness

Eyes
____Watery eyes
____Itchy eyes
____Swollen eyelids
____Sticky eyelids
____Dark circles
____Blurred vision

Weight
____Binge eating
____Cravings
____Excessive weight
____Compulsive eating
____Water retention
____Underweight

Joint & Muscles
____Pain in joints
____Arthritis
____Stiffness
____Limited movement
____Aches in muscles
____Feeling of weakness

Mouth & Throat

____Chronic coughing
____Gagging
____Often clear throat
____Sore throat
____Swollen tongue/lips
____Canker sores

Nose

____Stuffy nose
____Sinus problems
____Hay fever
____Sneezing attacks
____Excessive mucous

Head

____Headaches
____Faintness
____Dizziness
____Insomnia

Skin

____Acne
____Hives, rashes
____Hair loss
____Flushing/hot flashes
____Excessive sweating

Lungs

____Chest congestion
____Asthma, bronchitis
____Shortness of breath
____Difficulty breathing

Mind

____Poor memory
____Confusion
____Poor concentration
____Stuttering/ stammering
____Learning disabilities

Other

____Irregular heartbeat
____Rapid heartbeat
____Chest pains
____Frequent illness
____Frequent urination
____Genital itch

Bibliography

- Alun Jones, V. et al, Food intolerance: a major factor in the pathogenesis of irritable bowel syndrome, Lancet II, November 1982.
- Anderson, JA, Milk, eggs and peanuts: food allergies in children, Am Fam Physician, October 1987.
- Atherton DJ, Sewell M, Sothill JF et al, A double-blind controlled crossover trial of an antigen avoidance diet in atopic eczema, Lancet, February 25, 1978.
- Baraniuk, JN. Et al, (Non-IgE) Rhinitis symptoms in chronic fatigue syndrome, Ann Allergy Asthma Immunol, October 1998.
- Barau, E; Dupont, C, Modification of intestinal permeability during food provocation procedures in pediatric irritable bowel syndrome, Journal of Ped. Gastro. And Nutr, 1990.
- Barnes RMR Harvey MM Blears J et al, IgG Subclass of Human Serum Antibodies Reactive with Dietary Proteins, Int Archs Allergy appl. Immun, 1986.
- Bentley SJ, Pearson DJ, Rix KJB, Food hypersensitivity in IBS, Lancet II, August 1983.
- Bluestone ChD, Eustachian tube function and allergy in otitis media, Pediatrics, May 1978.
- Boris, M & Mandel, F, Foods and additives are common causes of the attention deficit hyperactive disorder in children, Annals of Allergy May 1994
- Carter, CM et al., Effects of a few food diet in attention deficit disorder, Archives of Disease in Children 1993
- Chandra RK, Five-year follow-up of high-risk infants with family history of allergy who were exclusively breastfed or fed partial whey hydrolysate, soy and conventional cow's milk formulas, Journal of Pediatric Gastro & Nutrition, April 1997.
- Chandra RK, Five-year follow-up of high-risk infants with family history of allergy who were exclusively breastfed or fed partial whey

hydrolysate, soy and conventional cow's milk formulas, J Pediatr Gastroenterol Nutr, April 1997.

- Chinnery PF et al, CSF antigliadin antibodies and the Ramsay Hunt syndrome, Neurology, October 1987.
- Ciacci, C. et al, Depressive symptoms in adult celiac disease, Scand J Gastroenterol, March 1998.
- JD, Identification of allergic factors in middle ear effusions, Ann Otol Rhinol Laryngol, 1976.
- Cohen GA Hartman F Hamburger RN et al, Severe Anemia and chronic Bronchitis associated with a Markedly Elevated Specific IgG to Cow's Milk Protein, Annals of Allergy, July 1985.
- Corvaglia, L. et al, Depression in adult untreated celiac subjects: diagnosis by the pediatrician, Am J Gastroentero, March 1999.
- Cronin, CC, Shanahan, F, Insulin-dependent diabetes mellitus and celiac disease, Lancet, April 12, 1997.
- Darlington LG, Ramsy NW, Mansfield JR, Placebo-controlled, blind study of dietary manipulation therapy in rheumatoid arthritis, Lancet, February 1986.
- Davison HM, The role of food sensitivity in nasal allergy, Ann Allergy, September 1951.
- Derebery, MJ; Berliner, KI, Allergy for the otologist. External canal to inner ear, Otolaryngol Clin North Am, February 1998.
- Derlacki EL, Food sensitization as a cause of perennial nasal allergy, Ann Allergy, November 1955.
- Deufemia P et al, Abnormal intestinal permeability in children with autism, Acta Paediatr, September 1986.
- Egger J, Carter BA, Soothill and Wilson, Oligoantigenic treatment of children with epilepsy and migraine, Journal of Pediatrics, January 1989.

- Egger J, Carter CM, Wilson J et al, Is migraine food allergy? A double-blind controlled trial of oligoantigenic diet treatment, Lancet II, October 1983.
- Egger, J et al., Controlled trial of oligoantigenic treatment of the hyperkinetic syndrome, The Lancet, March 9, 1985 and May 9, 1992.
- Egger, J et al., Food allergy and asthma, Annals of Allergy, December 1988.
- Farah DA, Calder I, Benson L, Mackenzie JF, Specific food intolerance: its place as a cause of gastrointestinal symptoms, Gut 1985.
- Finn, R, Food allergy-fact or fiction: a review, J R Soc Med, September 1982.
- Gerrard JW, Familial recurrent rhinorrhea and bronchitis due to cow's milk, JAMA, November 1966.
- Haddad, Vetter, Friedman, Samz, Brunner, Detection and kinetics of antigen-specific IgE and IgG immune complexes in food allergy, Annal of Allergy, August 1993.
- Hadley, JA, Evaluation and management of allergic rhinitis, Med Clin North Am, January 1999.
- Hamilton S. Dixon, MD, Treatment of delayed food allergy based on specific immunoglobulin G RAST testing, Otolaryngology Head and Neck Surgery, July 2000.
- Hammer H, Provocation with cow's milk and cereals in atopic dermatitis, Acta Derm Venereol (Stockh), 1977.
- Haugen, MA. Et al., A pilot study of the effect of an elemental diet in the management of rheumatoid arthritis, Clin Exp Rheumatol, 1994.
- Hurst, DS, Allergy management of refractory serous otitis media, Otolaryngol Head Neck Surg, June 1990.
- Iacono G et al, Persistent cow's milk protein intolerance (asthma, eczema, rhinitis) in infants: the changing faces of the same disease, Clin Exp Allergy, July 1998.

- Iacono G. et al, Persistent cow's milk protein intolerance (asthma, eczema, rhinitis) in infants: the changing faces of the same disease, Clin Exp Allergy, July 1998
- Jewell DP, Truelove SC, Reaginic hypersensitivity in ulcerative colitis, Gut 1972.
- Kahn A., et al, Milk intolerance in children with persistent sleeplessness: a prospective double-blind crossover evaluation, Pediatrics, October 1989.
- Kaplan, SJ et al., Dietary replacement in preschool-aged hyperactive boys, Pediatrics, January 1989
- Kemeny RD Urbanek R Amlot PL et al, Sub-class of IgG in allergic disease, I IgG subclass antibodies in immediate and non-immediate food allergy, Clinical Allergy, 1986.
- Kitts D. et al, Adverse reactions to food constituents: allergy, intolerance and auto-immunity, Can J Physiol Pharmacol, April 1987.
- Mansfield LE, Vaughan TR, Waller SF, Haverly RW, Ting S, Food Allergy and adult migraine: double-blind mediator confirmation of an allergic etiology, Ann Allergy, August 1985.
- Marshall, Attention deficit disorder and allergy: A neurochemical model of the relationship between illnesses, Psychology Bulletin. 1989
- Matsumoto, P et al., Markedly high eosinophilia and an elevated serum IL-5 level in an infant with cow milk allergy (induced anaphylaxis), Annals of Allergy, Asthma & Immunology, March 1999.
- Mendall, MA; Kumar D, Antibiotic use, childhood affluence (atopy) and irritable bowel syndrome (IBS), Eur J Gastroenterol Hepatol, 1998.
- Merrett J Peatfield RC Rose F Clifford et al, Food related antibodies in headache patients, Journal of Neurology, Neurosurgery and Psychiatry, 1983.
- Monro J, Carini C, Brostoff J, Migraine is a food-allergic disease, Lancet II, September 29, 1984.

- Morgan JE, Daul CB, Lehrer SB, The relationships among shrimp-specific IgG subclass antibodies and immediate adverse reactions to shrimp challenge, J Allergy Clin Immunol, September 1990.
- Niggemann, B. et al, Outcome of double-blind, placebo-controlled food challenge tests in 107 children with atopic dermatitis, Clin Exp Allergy, January 1999.
- November, E et al., Anaphylaxis in children: clinical and allergologic features, Pediatrics, April 1998.
- Nsouli TM et al, Role of food allergy in serous otitis media, Ann Allergy, September 1994.
- Ogle KA, Bullock JD, Children with allergic rhinitis and/or bronchial asthma treated with an elimination diet: a five-year follow-up, Ann Allergy, May 1980.
- Paganelli R Pallone F Montano S et al, Isotypic Analysis of Antibody Response to a Food Antigen in Inflammatory Bowel Disease, Int Archs Allergy appl. Immun, 1985.
- Panush RS, Stroud RM, Webster EM, Food-induced (allergic) arthritis. Inflammatory arthritis exacerbated by milk, Arthritis Rheum, February 1986.
- Pellegrino, M. et al, Untreated celiac disease and attempted suicide, Lancet, September 1995.
- Petitpierre, M et al, Irritable bowel syndrome and hypersensitivity to food, Annals of Allergy, June 1985.
- Rafei A, Peters S, Harris N, and Bellani J, Food allergy and food-specific IgG measurement, Annals of Allergy, February 1989.
- Ragnarsson G; Bodemar G, Pain is temporally related to eating but not to defecation in the irritable bowel syndrom (IBS). Patients' description of diarrhea, constipation and symptom variation during a prospective 6-week study, Eur J Gastroenterol Hepatol, May 1998.

- Rebuffat, E. et al, Difficulty in initiating and maintaining sleep associated with cow's milk allergy in infants, Sleep, April 1987.
- Roberts DL et al, Atopic features inulcerative colitis, Lancet, June 10, 1978.
- Rowe AH, Rowe A Jr, Perennial nasal allergy due to food sensitization, J Asthma Res, December 1965.
- Rowe AH, Young EJ, Bronchial asthma due to food allergy alone in 95 patients, JAMA, March 1959.
- Sampson HA, Role of immediate food hypersensitivity in the pathogenesis of atopic dermatis, J Allergy Clin Immunol, May 1983.
- Sampson HA, Jolie PL, Increased plasma histamine concentrations after food challenges in children with atopic dermatitis, New England Journal of Medicine, August 9, 1984.
- Schmidt, M Floch, MH, Food Hypersensitivity and the Irritable Bowel Syndrome, Am J of Gastroenterology, January 1992.
- Scott, FW. Et al, Milk and Type I Diabetes: Examining the evidence and broadening the focus, Diabetes Care, April 1986.
- Scott, FW. Et al, Potential mechanisms by which certain foods promote or inhibit the development of spontaneous diabetes in BB rats: dose, timing, early effects on islet area, and switch in infiltrate from Th1 to Th2 cells, Diabetes, April 1987.
- Stefanini, GF Prati, E Albini MC et al, Oral Disodium Chromoglycate Treatment of Irritable Bowel Syndrome: An Open Study on 101 subjects with Diarrheic Type (Comment: Cromoglycate), Am J of Gastroenterology, January 1992.
- Straus, SE. et al, Allergy and the chronic fatigue syndrome, J Allergy Clin Immunol, May 1988.
- van de Laar, MA, Food intolerance in rheumatoid arthritis II. Clinical and histological aspects, Ann Rheum Dis, March 1992.

- van de Laar, MA; van der Korst, JK, Food intolerance in rheumatoid arthritis. A double blind controlled trial of the clinical effects of elimination of milk allergens and azo dyes, Ann Rheum Dis, March 1992.
- Vitoria JC, Camarero C, Sojo A et al, Enteropathy related to fish, rice and chicken, Arch Dis Child, 1982.
- Wagner, WO, Angioedema: frightening and frustrating, Cleveland Clinic Journal of Medicine, April 1999.
- Wüthrich, B, Food-induced cutaneous adverse reactions, Allergy, 1998.
- Zetterstrom O, Food and asthma II, Eur J Respir Dis, 1984.